OUR WISDOM YEARS

absolutely unique questions of our lives. This is a book best used by lingering with it, not rushing through—a book of questions each of us might ponder in the silence of the heart until we hear the response of the still small voice within."

—STEVE ZEMMELMAN, MSW, PhD, Jungian Analyst and
Associate Clinical Professor, Department of Psychiatry,
University of California at San Francisco

"*Our Wisdom Years* offers a gentle, thorough, and soulful way into life's deepest and most challenging stage—the path of aging. Although he is an accomplished psychologist with many stories to tell (including, most wonderfully, his own), Dr. Garfield writes like a gentle friend. This book is a guide for the journey into 'the glorious mess of self,' at a time in life when self is most poignant. Full of questions to ponder, exercises to engage, and thoughts to contemplate, *Our Wisdom Years* will help you foster 'your own relationship to eternity.'"

—NORMAN FISCHER, poet, Zen priest, author,
The World Could Be Otherwise: Imagination and the Bodhisattva Path

"*Our Wisdom Years* arrived shortly after I turned eighty-two. I've lived a fulfilling life, but am all too aware of my age-related declines and struggling with them. The book is so helpful! I'm underlining most of it. I haven't done that since college! Garfield's understanding of my and others' transitions, understanding from the heart as well as the head, is opening possibilities and easing transitions. Thank you!"

—CHARLES T. TART, PhD, Emeritus Professor of Psychology,
University of California at Davis and
author of *The Secret Science of the Soul*

"Charles Garfield has one of our biggest hearts and wisest minds, and I am privileged to call him a mentor of mine. *Our Wisdom Years,* a true masterpiece, is a marvelously rich mix of wise counsel and comforting possibility for all of us who are feeling the pull of our later years. It is a profound reflection on aging that offers all those of a certain age the guidance we'll need to navigate later life with soul and satisfaction. This is a book of immense honesty, courage, and grace. You'll be delighted that you've moved it to the top of your reading list."

—KAUSHIK ROY, executive director of Shanti Project:
Enhancing the Health, Quality of Life, and Well-Being
of People with Terminal, Life-Threatening,
or Disabling Illnesses or Conditions

"Charles Garfield is one of our most open-hearted and intelligent teachers on the subject of aging. His latest book, *Our Wisdom Years*, is an exciting and illuminating look at the potential we all have to live later life with wisdom, compassion, and courage. This book stands out in its genre as a beacon of guidance and generosity, a genuine gift to all those who have entered their wisdom years. I enjoyed and learned an enormous amount from this work of Dr. Garfield. You'll be extremely glad you've read *Our Wisdom Years*."

—JIM SANTUCCI, executive director of Kara: Grief Support
for Children, Teens, Families, and Adults

"Once again, Dr. Charles Garfield offers us a deep work of soul with a book exploring the wisdom, joy, and resilience that can be found with aging. Garfield tenderly invites the reader to consider nine tasks, empowering one to deeply consider the growth and healing available to us all when we 'allow ourselves to accept the true gifts of age that bring us into our own.' As I stand firmly in midlife, I find the sacred storytelling in this work provoking and challenging. This marvelous book allows me to consider how I'd like my own 'wisdom years' to unfold."

—DR. GINA BELTON, PhD, Professor of Psychology at Saybrook University

OUR WISDOM YEARS

CHARLES GARFIELD, PhD

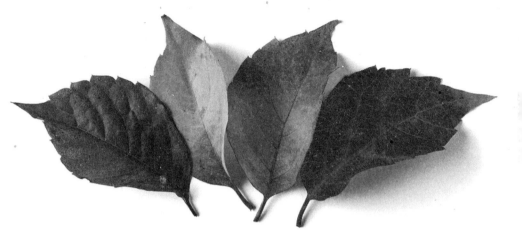

Our

WISDOM
YEARS

Growing Older with Joy, Fulfillment,
Resilience, and No Regrets

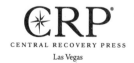

CENTRAL RECOVERY PRESS

Las Vegas

AURORA PUBLIC LIBRARY

Central Recovery Press (CRP) is committed to publishing exceptional materials addressing addiction treatment, recovery, and behavioral healthcare topics.

For more information, visit www.centralrecoverypress.com.

Publisher: Central Recovery Press
          3321 N. Buffalo Drive
          Las Vegas, NV 89129

25 24 23 22 21 20   1 2 3 4 5

Library of Congress Cataloging-in-Publication Data

Names: Garfield, Charles A., author.
Title: Our wisdom years : growing older with joy, fulfillment, resilience,
    and no regrets / Charles Garfield.
Description: Las Vegas, NV : Central Recovery Press, 2020. | Summary: "In
    Our Wisdom Years, Dr. Charles Garfield skillfully and practically guides
    readers through nine tasks that can transform the struggles of aging,
    bringing fulfillment, joy, and serenity"-- Provided by publisher.
Identifiers: LCCN 2019054966 (print) | LCCN 2019054967 (ebook) | ISBN
    9781949481181 (hardcover) | ISBN 9781949481198 (ebook)
Subjects: LCSH: Older people--Life skills guides. | Aging--Social aspects.
Classification: LCC HQ1061 .G365 2020 (print) | LCC HQ1061 (ebook) | DDC
    305.26--dc23
LC record available at https://lccn.loc.gov/2019054966
LC ebook record available at https://lccn.loc.gov/2019054967

Photo of Charles Garfield by Stu Selland. Used with permission.

Every attempt has been made to contact copyright holders. If copyright holders have not been properly acknowledged please contact us. Central Recovery Press will be happy to rectify the omission in future printings of this book.

Publisher's Note: This book contains general information about aging and related matters. The information contained herein is not medical advice. This book is not an alternative to medical advice from your doctor or other professional healthcare provider.

Our books represent the experiences and opinions of their authors only. Every effort has been made to ensure that events, institutions, and statistics presented in our books as facts are accurate and up-to-date. To protect their privacy, the names of some of the people, places, and institutions in this book may have been changed.

Cover design and interior by Marisa Jackson.

TO ALL THOSE KINDRED SPIRITS OF
A CERTAIN AGE WHO ARE DISCOVERING
GENUINE FULFILLMENT IN LATER LIFE,
AND TO CINDY SPRING, WHOSE ENDURING LOVE
ENABLES ME TO BE AMONG THOSE FORTUNATE ONES.

CONTENTS

EXERCISES & PRACTICES

AUTHOR'S NOTE

I wasn't taking notes while I lived most of the experiences described in *Our Wisdom Years*. In fact, in many cases, I had no idea I would be writing this book at all. Although I'm now seventy-five years old, my memory of real-life situations didn't seem to fail me as I relate the stories I tell and describe the people I've met. All in all, they reflect my current recollection of what we experienced recently and, at times, years ago.

All quoted dialogue and comments are reconstructed from memory, not from transcriptions. I've tried to be true to the spirit and substance of what happened and to give an honest depiction of these experiences and events. Some of the people who share their stories are identified by their real names, but the names of many other older people, family, and friends have been changed, as have many identifying details of their situations. Also, certain individuals are composites. Any similarity to persons living or dead resulting from these changes is completely coincidental and unintentional.

INTRODUCTION

Across Japan for a couple of short weeks every spring, whole communities gather under the pale pink clouds of blossoms that fill the cherry trees. It's a celebration of beauty made all the more precious because it's so brief. The blossoms might glow for only a week or two before they disappear in huge flurries, leaving the branches bare. The falling of the blossoms is poignant and treasured. *Hanafubuki* it's called—flower (*hana*) snowstorm (*fubuki*).

There's a bittersweet quality to those celebrations and their symbolism that I recognize from my own life. In a most poetic way, gathering under the trees as the petals drift down is a way not only of drinking in the spectacle of life at its peak but of acknowledging how short that time is and how evanescent our days.

I know that well, after many years of working with the dying. Physical beauty fades. Death comes. It's the interval in between that bedevils us, the stretch of life when try as we might, we can't keep the bloom of youth pasted to the branches anymore, and the givens that have defined us fall away. We thought that we would always be the strong one, the vital one, the contributor, the dutiful son or rebellious daughter; time somehow wouldn't touch us. And then comes our own flower snowstorm.

Like many people I know, I was at the end of my forties when I began getting the first gut-deep messages that my hold on invulnerability was beginning to slip, and time was carrying my whole world that much closer to its end. My father, always healthy, developed an aggressive, fatal cancer. In my late fifties, so did my best friend. A few years later, my mother was gone, too. Then the arthritis that had been progressing in my hip unnoticed, probably for years, became debilitating overnight and it was hard for me to walk. As my sixties progressed, there was more news of sick friends. More of loved ones who'd died. I got steady reminders of how urgent it was to live my life to the full, yet the things I had always done didn't seem satisfying anymore. Anytime I thought of how quickly time seemed to be passing, I wanted to fill each moment with passion, but strangely, I couldn't imagine how.

Such times, for many of us, are an initiation we don't know how to navigate, a shift that carries us toward unmapped territory. We don't know how to let go of who we were in our youth and earlier adulthood, even as the trappings and constants of our old identities flutter to the ground. We don't yet know that the only way to experience the deep beauty, growth, and freedom of our later years is to release the parts of our lives that no longer fit.

When we are willing to enter the darkness of this unknown time and slowly let our eyes and souls adjust, bright constellations of meaning—and a tremendous sense of awe—become palpable to us, showing us who we are becoming, who we are large enough to be.

Too often, though, we're afraid to explore. We don't realize that in this new place—informed by loss and also by astonishing joy—we have the opportunity to claim our authentic self. But this is what my life and work have taught me: if we take the risk of shedding outworn roles and expanding our definition of ourselves, we can let our souls lead us to the full expression of who we are, the self we were always meant to be. That is the promise that belongs to us as we grow toward wisdom.

This book is a guide to the journey.

——— ———

Allowing ourselves to accept the true gifts of age brings us into our own, and it can open us to a kind of peace we've likely never known. But I learned that only reluctantly. Like many people, I didn't want anything to do with the changes that come as we grow older—they just weren't for me.

Without thinking too much about it, I had always assumed that once I became an adult, I would carry on with the same sorts of ambitions, goals, and desires for the rest of my life. Yes, I might slow down, but I assumed that I'd work at "aging successfully"—that is, with as little evidence of aging as possible. There was no reason to think I wouldn't stay essentially healthy, active, youthful, and successful for the rest of my life. I figured I might slow down some, maybe take things at three-quarter speed in my nineties, but even then, I imagined I'd be the same as always.

What shocked me, as I absorbed the losses I faced in my fifties and sixties, was how much they changed me. I began to realize that I *wasn't* the same, inside or out.

I can pinpoint the moment when the business of aging got personal. I was in an exercise class—not an over-the-top boot camp, but a gentle session focused on body alignment. I was lying on my back, stretching my leg over to one side. Simple, especially for someone like me; I'd been working out since I was in my teens and I still went to the gym regularly to do a weights routine. I could look in the mirror and see that I was good as ever, maybe not the committed body builder I'd been in my twenties, but plenty flexible and fit. If anyone wanted proof that sixty is the new forty, they could just snap my picture.

But I was new to the class, and maybe I pushed a little too hard trying to keep up with (or—okay—*impress*) the people around me. I tended to do that then. During the session, I thought I was doing fine, but when I stood up, my hip was out of whack and I felt a sharp pain when I walked that didn't subside. I limped out the door, thinking I must've pulled something. When I was still limping a week later, I went into "I can solve this" mode. I got a massage. Then I tried Rolfing. And yoga. And every kind of bodywork and alternative therapy you can imagine. Nothing helped.

Simply walking turned into a painful chore, and I could scarcely go a block without needing to sit down. Finally, after months of struggle, I went for an ultrasound and X-ray. That's when I got the news that I had arthritis and needed a hip replacement.

What stunned me was how suddenly everything changed. I woke up the morning of my fateful class and launched into the day much as I had for years—with a to-do list, a full calendar of activities, and people to meet. That familiar life was a race I ran every day, thriving, accomplishing things, in my prime. But by nightfall, the smallest step was difficult. For the first time, I felt old.

That's often how the fact of our aging breaks into our consciousness. A body part stops working. The barrier that seemed to keep us invulnerable to loss or injury gets flimsy. Routines that used to satisfy us feel empty. A shock to the system wakes us up or tries to.

The message being transmitted is simple and neutral: "You're changing. Time for something new." But we don't tend to read it that way. It's common instead to imagine that we've started on a horrific narrative of decline in which we lose everything—beauty, functionality, independence, health, dignity—and then we die. The moral of that story is: just don't get old. Fight off aging! Don't even *say* the word.

I was inclined to do that myself. If not for a quirk of my psyche, I'm fairly certain that I would've signed up for the hip replacement immediately, given myself a short while to recuperate, and then taken up marathon running or done something equally extreme to prove that I was once more "the new forty" and invincible.

But fortunately for me, I was crazily, irrationally afraid of going under the knife. I was certain that I would be the one who would die on the operating table during this common, low-risk surgery, or maybe I'd wake up crippled for life. So, I waited four years before having my hip replaced and "getting my life back."

Those slowed-down years were a pivotal period when I began to accept that I was not exempt from the physical, psychological, and spiritual evolution that wants to transform us in later life. I'd been in the honeymoon period—that stretch through our fifties and early sixties when it's still possible to blink away the different, older version of ourselves that's beginning to come into focus. But forced to adjust both my pace and my plans, I let that new person, the self I was becoming at sixty-four, emerge. My old life didn't quite fit anymore. I was restless, and my hip problem felt like the least of it. During the frequent pauses that now punctuated my days, I let myself acknowledge how exhausting it had been to keep myself in constant motion, staying on a path chosen by someone much different, decades before. What would I choose if I were setting out afresh? I thought about roads not taken.

Slowly, I found myself relaxing my grip on many of the beliefs and attitudes that had defined me. Of course good health was and is important to me, but my life wasn't ruined when I lost the speed and strength and "perfection" I used to have. Looking in the mirror at the gym at an older guy with a bit of a paunch gazing back at me, I smiled at him instead of looking away with a sigh of regret. Having a bad hip had forced me to be gentle with myself, for the first time in my life. Kinder. I understood in a new way that there was more to me than my body.

Perhaps most surprising, I didn't feel as compulsively driven as I had before; quite a turnabout for a guy who had literally written the book *Peak Performers*, a 1980s guide to success and achievement. How people got the most satisfaction from their working lives had always interested me, and I'd frequently counseled them to "be sure the ladder you're climbing is against the right wall." But now a new thought burbled up: "There doesn't have to be a ladder."

The prospect made me smile—and then it stopped me cold. What would that mean? What would I be without the push to do more, improve, always be productive? Would I simply go soft? I had always lived by *Faster, Stronger, Higher* and *Good, Better, Best*. But I noticed that words like *deeper* and *clearer* and *truer* resonated with me now. They seemed to be more concerned with inner states than outer ones. The nagging, pushy, "Do more!" voice in my mind got quieter, and I liked the calm that brought.

It took much searching to understand what was going on. I was moving from one stage of life to another, from adulthood into the distinct, post-adult stage of later life—the profound passage that lets us complete our lives, as in make them *whole*.

It's only in the past couple of decades that the post-adult period has gotten much notice in America. (Some call it *elderhood*, but I like the simplicity of "later life.") Psychologists like Harry Moody began talking about "conscious aging," seeing it as a path to a stage of development in which we can grow beyond the ambitions and desires that shape our earlier lives. It's not an easy, or even a required path, he pointed out. It's shaped by spirit, not success.

As adults, we want control, competence, and mastery, the sorts of things I used to teach people in my books and lectures on success. And who wouldn't want to be competent, to excel at something important to them, to set goals and reach them? We're immersed in the language of success, self-mastery, and self-confidence, and it's not something we tend to question as we get older. Why should we? We've been working at this our whole lives and we want to stand out, not disappear.

But now, in these later decades of life, our desires are different. There can be yet another iteration of ourselves, a kind of Self 4.0, that follows our incarnations as child, adolescent, and adult. This version of who we are takes shape around the same core we've always had. But now, if we're willing to let it, that core becomes more visible. It emerges, elegant and elemental, the way the dark boughs of a cherry tree do after their blossoms have been lifted away. That's one of the primary missions of these later decades of life: to reveal and revel in our true nature, which may have been hidden or eclipsed while we were doing our duty, performing roles chosen long ago, meeting others' needs.

As we drop old ways of being, we become ourselves, only more so—more inclined to do what makes us feel most alive, more willing to bring our desires into the light, more curious about what our lives have meant, more open to things that bring us joy, more able to say yes to what has meaning for us, and we begin to let go of what doesn't.

This period of life can be our "someday"—as in, "Someday I'll finally let myself expand into the person I was always meant to be." It isn't a matter of trying to be who we think we *should* be or striving toward some external ideal so we can follow someone else's recipe for "being a better person." This shift is about gravitating toward the vastness that's always been inside us, calling to us to take a chance on ourselves and *live*.

What I've just described may sound selfish or self-absorbed, especially to people who've borne or still bear heavy responsibility for others and are in the habit of pushing their own desires to the background. But later life is actually a time of *interdependence*, when we clearly see the value of sharing ourselves and our gifts with those who mean the most to us in an open exchange of the heart, sometimes offering and supporting, sometimes leaning and receiving. It's also a period when we are drawn to deepen our connections to and love for other people, savoring them and our time together.

Because this stretch of life leads all the way to the end, there's another mission that gains urgency as our years pass: we're drawn to develop a relationship with what will outlast us and the parts of ourselves that will live on. We are, in a sense, developing a relationship with eternity. That begins with considering our legacy, what we want to leave behind, what we hope someone will carry into the world for us when we're no longer here. This can be a time when the dominant theme of our lives becomes *unity*, when we realize as never before that we are spirit as well as flesh, and finally find the peace and balance that come from embracing the eternal.

I know this is not how most people think about the years after sixty or seventy. It's easy to stay locked in the perspective of adulthood, asking, "How much am I achieving? How well am I competing? How young do I look?" But if we slow down and listen to our souls, we notice that the questions are changing. Instead of anxiously asking, "Do I have what it takes to compete?" we allow ourselves to wonder: "Do I have what it takes to *lead a fulfilling life*?"

In later life, the drive to keep moving, keep accomplishing, begins to seem less interesting than the understandings we find in solitude or the moments of awe we feel in nature or as we hold a new grandchild. What we want more than success or things are loving relationships—an intimacy with the eternal and our deep, wild selves—and a life built around *that*.

We get glimpses of these rearranged priorities when we're confronted with a loss like the death of a parent or as we sit with a friend who's going through chemo. What matters most—to them and us— isn't whether we're getting wrinkles, chasing some kind of recognition, or "staying young and active"; it's what our lives have meant, who we are to each other, what we love, and what parts of ourselves will live on in each other or eternity. What matters, urgently, is what we make of the life we have right now.

The particularly tough thing, I've noticed, is that many of us don't know how to keep this understanding as time passes. We get a taste of what is most important and sense how crucial it is to *keep* our focus there, but we quickly whistle past the awareness. We do our best to go back to succeeding, achieving, doing—"getting on with life" as our adult selves (and the world around us) insist we should— instead of walking through the gate toward our deeper selves and centering our lives around what we *love*.

All too often, as I sat at the bedside of people with just months or days to live, I wished that they had been able to explore much earlier what was truly important to them and to fill their days up with it, rather than scrambling in their final moments to make peace with their regrets, their unanswered questions, their unspoken words of forgiveness and gratitude, and their unlived dreams. The chapters to come will help you begin today to take the risk of being fully alive in later life, right here, right now. I can't offer a 1-2-3 linear formula because realizing our truest selves is an unfolding that will take the rest of our lives. Instead, I've outlined three levels of exploration for this time of life and drawn a path through them, illustrated with my story and the stories of many others. The route is winding, and I urge you to spend time with what calls to you in the moment and to linger with any practice, exercise, or chapter that speaks to you.

The first section of this book, "Tuning in to the Voice of Wisdom," provides an overview of the themes you'll be exploring in greater depth as we go on. You'll get the most from the book if you read and play with the first three chapters in order. You'll meet inner advisers who can help you along the way, open up space where you can get to know yourself as you are now, and discover ways to activate joy.

The second section, "Seeing Your Life through Wisdom's Eyes and Heart," is devoted to looking inward through three distinct lenses: life review, forgiveness, and gratitude. These, not coincidentally, are the urgent themes of the very end of life, the places where people seek and find meaning and peace. Taking the time to explore them now will allow you to move through your wisdom years with energy, insight, and joy.

The final section, "Opening to the Eternal," turns your focus outward: first toward the world and your new role in it, then toward the people and beings you love, and finally toward the Mystery of eternity. This is soul-focused territory that becomes ever more compelling as time passes.

The nine Tasks of Transformation you'll find in these chapters offer a vision of growth and expansion in a time we tend to associate with decline and, taken together, they create a solid foundation from which to navigate all the changes and challenges ahead. They'll center you in what brings you most alive and help you cultivate a sense of vision, resilience, and equanimity that you can count on no matter what.

I've used these tasks as a guide for students in classes on how to follow our callings and our untamed nature in our wisdom years, and we frequently begin by considering May Sarton's words:

Now I become myself. It's taken
Time, many years and places;
I have been dissolved and shaken,
Worn other people's faces . . .

As adults, we make plans, check things off our lists, and keep ourselves advancing even as we cling to the safety of what we know. But in the wisdom years, we keep *listening* in the knowledge that there's no end to the call and response of the spirit, no end to being dissolved and shaken, right up to the last breath.

Working with the dying and with people who, like me, were reluctant to accept the gifts that come with age, has taught me that there's tremendous freedom in living out our lives with curiosity, a sense of humor, and open eyes—not fearful, but aware that our time is short, and our bodies will break down. We cannot stay the same as we ever were, nor would we want to.

The beautiful paradox of growing older is that none of the gifts of age are available without the kind of loss that forces us to confront mortality in a way we can't deny. In the face of loss, we're changed and expanded by truths that come from the heart, not the mind. We learn that we're part of something much larger than we are; that love and kindness matter most of all. The wisdom that allows us to value and *live by* those truths can't be reduced to slogans like "When life hands you lemons, make lemonade!" It sounds and feels more like what Naomi Shihab Nye writes in her poem "Kindness":

Before you know what kindness really is
you must lose things,
feel the future dissolve in a moment
like salt in a weakened broth . . .

Before you know kindness as the deepest thing inside,
you must know sorrow as the other deepest thing. . . .

Then it is only kindness that makes sense anymore . . .

Wisdom isn't for the "immortal," the untouched, the ones who tie their worth to the surface. It requires letting the petals fall to reveal the true shape of the much larger self that's been hidden inside us, the profound but simple truths of life, the exquisite Mystery that surrounds us.

Life is calling us to this—to our wisdom years. I invite you to say yes.

PART ONE

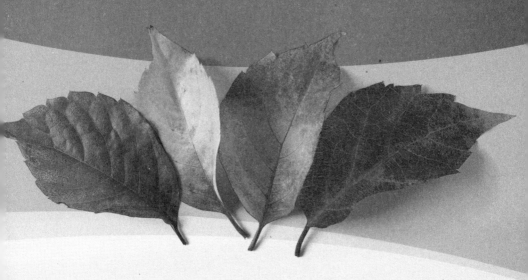

Tuning in
TO THE
Voice of Wisdom

CHAPTER ONE

THE FIRST TASK

Convene an Inner Council of Advisers

S omething inside you is pressing to be born.

It's rich with the potential you've carried inside for years but haven't fully nurtured into being.

This new surge of energy that wants to reshape your life may show itself first as a daydream that makes you well up with excitement or joy. It could drift into view as the memory of a path not taken, a dream or talent you put on the shelf because it wasn't "practical."

Some of us feel it as a longing that keeps returning: "I'd love to . . ." "I wish I could . . ." "It would feel so good to just . . ." Or it may appear simply as a feeling that "there's so much more to me than what I've let myself be so far."

The face and form of this desire may not be clear to you yet. It may be no more than a murmur at the back of your mind, a sense of restlessness or boredom or hope. But it's urgent to seek it out and to devote yourself to its care. Answering its call—which beckons you to wisdom and fulfillment—is the mission of later life.

It's not a given that you will hear that call and respond. I'm aware that it could seem almost absurd to think of yourself as being "pregnant" now with a hunger for something deep and new. Here in the home stretch of life, a lot of us thought we were supposed to be enjoying the fruits of the effort we poured into earning the success, mastery, and ease that come with years of devotion to building our lives and livelihoods. We've had our children, literal and creative, and now, in the laid-back "golden years," we might've thought we had things figured out and were done with the work of discovering who we are and how best to live.

Such assumptions are prevalent in part because the possibility of later-life transformation has been a fairly well-kept secret in our culture, which tends to insist that any real potential for growth is used up by the end of adulthood. It's actually a fascinating trap. Any diminished interest in what's always consumed us—jobs, assigned roles, success, other people's priorities—is taken as evidence of our woeful decline. But the startling truth is that with lifespans lengthening, we're now spending roughly a *third* of our lives in our post-adult years where our old passions and preoccupations don't satisfy us in the same way anymore. If we let ourselves, we have a chance to grow in new directions and to savor what brings us bliss. We've been handed an invaluable prize but because it comes with an AARP card, we frequently don't want to take it. At the cusp of the opportunity of a lifetime, we've too often been brainwashed into believing we'd prefer to stay the same as we've always been.

When the idea of birthing or liberating a new vision of ourselves at age sixty or seventy or eighty comes up in my workshops on later life, there's often a bit of incredulity at first, even among those who are quite self-aware. Enticing as growth and fulfillment may sound, our first reaction is often some variation of: "I'm supposed to do *what?*"

We're finally at the point where we can dance like Fred Astaire through the familiar challenges we face, and suddenly someone's saying we need to do it backward, wearing heels? Isn't "discovering myself" for the young? Why complicate a life that's worked just fine, thanks to decades worth of effort? Why stumble? Why chase some old fantasy or silly pipe dream? Why screw things up?

As the voices of resistance build to a roar, it's supremely easy to talk ourselves out of our longings, and to stall at the threshold between who we've been as adults and all we could become in later life.

But if we can just disconnect from the momentum of our habits and routines and listen inwardly, there it is—a stubborn call to grow beyond who we've been. The desires speaking to us now can lead us to become someone different from the person we've so far allowed ourselves to be, someone less tamed by expectations and more reverent toward our deepest nature.

That's why the first task of transformation is to bring new voices, perspectives, and urgency into the discussion.

I'd like you to do that by consulting three inner advisers: Death, your Wise Self, and the Soul-Focused Adult inside you. The unique questions each of them will prompt you to ask about your life will help you take stock of where you are, where you've been, and what might be calling to you in your wisdom years. Throughout the book, these advisers will help you stay tethered to your most meaningful desires, encourage you to persist long enough to feel yourself change, and connect you with joy, even eternity. Consulting them and learning to rely on their guidance will open the door to the richness of later life.

The First Adviser: Death

Death may seem to be a bracing, even threatening choice for an adviser, but by the time we reach our sixties, or even our mid-fifties, it's no longer a stranger. It's likely that we've lost or begun to lose the older generation of our family and that an accident or disease has claimed someone in our circle.

As time passes, there's no escaping news of illness or loss in our conversations and social media feeds, and each time it comes close, we feel not only a pang of sadness but also a fresh zap that says, "Whoa! Death is real!" And we're not immune. As the Zen teacher Susan Murphy writes, "A time comes when it is no longer convincing to continue to live as if we had an eternity of time ahead of us."

And that being the case, Death prompts the question, "How will you use your precious, finite life?"

As we make a conscious effort to pause our habitual way of being and consider new ways forward into this stage of our lives, Death can act as the great awakener, disruptor, and pattern-breaker. It wants us to look again at our plans and calendars and ask: Does this still matter to me? If I knew I'd be gone in a month or a year or an hour, would this activity that seems so important be on the list of what I most need to do? What's *really* most meaningful?

The presence of Death provides a cold splash of clarity. But I don't suggest trying to hold onto that clarity by pelting yourself with a panicked "I'm going to die! I'm going to die! I'm going to die!" I think the most common response to such alarm is fear and a powerful desire to "get back to normal"—aka denial—or pretending that we are, and will always be, "as good as we ever were." It's more effective to keep Death at our shoulder by staying in conversation with the questions that it asks, its prompts that keep us awake to both the passage of time and the possibilities in each precious moment.

Looking Forward and Back at the Threshold to Later Life

As you stand at this threshold of life, accompanied by Death's questions, you might think of yourself as preparing to enter a fruitful night like the one that unfolds in *A Christmas Carol*, Dickens's classic story in which the ghosts of past, present, and future force Ebenezer Scrooge to review the choices he's made and see where his present trajectory might lead. If we let Death join us as we travel back in time, it's as though it challenges us to see the distinctive person we were early in life and who we've allowed that boy or girl to become. Death asks us to remember the seeds of potential entrusted to us, pointing to them as though they were part of a contract, and saying, "This is what you agreed to bring into the world. What have you done with it?"

Death gives us a preview of what our lives will become if we continue on without making any changes, ignoring the dreams and longings still unexpressed inside us. *This isn't a test run,* our own Ghost of the Future reminds us—*it's the real thing. Is this what you mean for your life to be?*

We'll do a careful life review farther on in the book. But you can begin to ask Death's questions now, slowly letting them interrupt your automatic responses and color your thinking, your choices. You can ask, and keep asking:

- What genuinely matters to me?
- Does *this* [grievance, activity, ritual, "thing I always do"] really matter anymore?
- What pettiness can I drop?
- What longings and risks and loves and promises to myself have I turned away from and at what cost?
- Will I let myself die without having lived?

A First Conversation with Death

I'd like to suggest a personal meditation that can be a way of tracing time and appreciating what's mattered to you in a way that gently invites in the perspective of Death.

You could do this anywhere, but if you can, take yourself to a place in nature that inspires you, a place where you can sit undisturbed with your thoughts. If you're lucky enough to be under a tree or near a garden, you'll probably be able to see the cycle of life around you, buds or blooms or fallen leaves, grass in shades of green and brown, birds resting and flying, stitching together the space of trees and sky. If you're in a park, you might find yourself watching the traffic of insects emerging from a crack in a sidewalk. Enjoy what flows around you for a while. Breathe it all in.

Then shift your attention to your hands. You might hold them in front of you or rest them on your lap, letting your thumbs trace the contours of the fingers beside them. Feel the softness or roughness of your skin and let one hand explore the other, the nails and tips of your fingers, rings you may have worn now for decades. Now turn both hands palm up and study them. Held this way it's possible that they look much the same as they have for decades. Fingers straight, palms plump and soft, or callused from some kind of labor. Even if arthritis or injury has sculpted knobs at your knuckles or time has left a tracery of veins in your fingers, you can feel the life in these hands.

Think about all your hands have done—the way they learned to tie shoelaces, hold a pencil, and cup clear running water to your mouth. Think of the way they reached for your mother when you were small, and how they've caressed and soothed and pulled to you so many people you've loved. Remember those people.

Think of the hammers or knitting needles or Frisbees or paintbrushes these hands have learned to guide, the notes they've typed, the laundry they've folded, the things they've carried and stroked and created. Perhaps they've made music or landed slaps or wiped away tears. Remember their power to heal and delight and connect and express.

A lifetime of sensory memories and training and love rests in these hands, which, as you see them in front of you now, hold so much possibility, so many gifts, so much bodily knowledge of how you have built your life. Linger over your memories of who these hands have touched, what they've made, how they've served.

Now turn your hands over and study them.

They may look far different than they did when you were young. Many of us can see the roundness of youth drained away from the backs of our hands to reveal the outlines of tendons, the clearer shapes of bones, and dark rivers of veins, the inside of us rising to the surface. Others may see the enlarged joints that we remember our parents or grandparents having as they tried to rub away their aches.

Your hands may be swollen or marked by hours in the sun and the way time erases the even coloring of youth and leaves its own collections of dots and blotches. Even if they are remarkably youthful, these are not the hands of a teenager, not the hands of the man or woman you were in your thirties. Seeing this side of our hands, the surface that faces outward, places us in the present moment, in the bodies that will carry us through later life. As you contemplate your hands now, appreciate all they've done, all they've yet to do. Let the years you see reflected in their physical form remind you, too, of how time keeps passing, even when it stands still in our minds. There will be a limit to how much we can bring into this world.

Let the two sides of your hands connect you with memory, possibility, time. Let them help you think about the side of yourself you turn to the world and the one that's softer, more hidden, closer to your core. And then allow Death to whisper its questions once again: *What will you do now with this precious, finite life? What really matters most?*

Listen for the answers that bubble up and be willing to keep listening long after you've heard the automatic and easy responses. Be willing to not know yet, but to keep asking. Throughout this book, you'll be disconnecting old habits and certainties so you can feel your way toward a vision of life that's a departure from what you've allowed yourself so far. One phase of life is ending; a new one is making its way to the surface. Making the most of this transition requires *taking your time* to discover what's true for you now.

Questions about Eternity

What questions do you have for Death? Often they revolve around the deep spiritual concerns that become urgent for us when we get to the end of our lives, and they begin to take on increasing importance as we step from adulthood into later life.

These are the *big* questions, the ones that can seem too vast to contemplate:

- Why am I here in this life? What am I here to do?
- Is there an afterlife? If so, what does it look like?
- Are we more than these bodies? Is there a nonmaterial part of myself, a soul? What would it mean if there is?
- What is my relationship with the eternal?

Death can't answer these questions for us with a lightning bolt or a thundering voice from the great beyond, but keeping its presence beside us—reminding us that we can't afford to wait any longer to enter the great mysteries of life—can help keep our focus on finding out what we truly believe.

Working with people who are in their dying time, I've seen repeatedly that when Death's questions remain unexamined until the very end of life, there's a desperate need to find the peace that comes from having a connection with a sense of the eternal that lies inside and beyond us—whatever we understand that to be.

We're fortunate now to have time to contemplate, question, and explore. Again, we won't rush the process. We'll address these questions directly toward the end of the book, allowing our relationship to them to slowly come into focus.

For now, just drop one of Death's questions into your mind and let it float there:

What am I here to do in this life?

The Second Adviser: The Wise Self

Even if you're like me and keep a plaster skull as a memento mori on your desk, it's not easy to stay with the stark questions and directives of Death and translate them into the everyday rhythms of human life. That's especially true when we begin to feel restless and unsatisfied with the roles that have defined us or see them crumbling as children leave home and longtime work ends. The question, "Who am I now?" can catch us without a clear answer, and we can feel as if we've been thrust into the space between trapezes where everything is up for grabs, with no assurances that we'll get a grip on this person we're becoming or that we'll land intact.

It's not a state we want to stay in for long. It's far easier to resist uncertainty by staying in motion, comforting ourselves with the familiar or distracting ourselves with a jam-packed roster of activities whose only virtue is that they keep us too busy to feel the confusion.

That's why it helps to seek support from a second adviser. Call it your wise, expanded self—the part of you that voices the wisdom you have at your core.

The Wise Self understands that the transition we're being asked to make in the last segment of our lives involves pivoting away from duty and toward joy. The mission of later life, your Wise Self will tell you, is not to strive for perfection, earn your right to keep existing, or work to "be a better person." Rather, the goal is to be the authentic, enlivened person you are when you're led not just by your mind but also by your heart and spirit.

What's truly important now? Pleasure, purpose, joy, and awe are the criteria your Wise Self will urge you to use as a filter for answering Death's questions about what really matters. Our time may be getting shorter, but time slows and deepens as we sink into each moment, immersed in what has meaning for us. Our sense of who we are can expand exponentially even as time contracts. We can come in contact with the eternal.

The realm of joy and the eternal isn't unknown territory. Starting at midlife, in our forties and fifties, many of us have awarenesses that seem like blessed accidents, which give a taste of what it's like to transcend everyday life and step into the world that lies beyond our egos. I think of a trip I took in my late forties to Mont Blanc. A friend invited me to climb a difficult trail, and though I was untrained and massively unprepared, I agreed to join him. It was only will, and a desire not to be shown up, that kept me from heading down after the first small rise, and somehow, I drove myself up and up.

I was sore, blistered, and spent when we finally reached our camp, and it took me a long while to pull my attention from my aching lungs and feet and look around. When I finally did, I was stunned to realize that we had gotten ourselves to a place of indescribable beauty. It was sunset, and I stood with my friend looking at the vast, deepening sky, the majestic peaks. "I'm one with all this," I realized. I knew with certainty that the expanse of awe that opened up inside me, so much larger than my body, was who I really am.

I replayed that scene again and again when I got home, struck by the way the most memorable part was not the achievement of climbing a mountain, but the wonder of being swallowed up by the beauty of that sunset. It was awe, not pride, which filled me up.

And then I got busy again—too busy for beauty, too distracted to be amazed. It took me many years to escape the grip of busy-ness and hear my Wise Self point out that the sense of expansion and elevation I'd found on the mountain was as close as the sky above my head and the sunset at the end of the street. Awe didn't need a mountaintop. It simply needed my willing presence.

It's easy to freeze up when Death asks, "What's your relationship to eternity?" Our minds can tangle us up in questions about religion and philosophy, heaven and hell. But the Wise Self reminds us that we already know the eternal and have stepped into it each time we've let ourselves be transported by love, beauty, awe, a sense of mystery, and experiences that have broadened our sense of reality. Now, in later life, we can devote ourselves to exploring this expansive realm so we can understand it from the inside and carry it with us.

Begin by asking the Wise Self's questions:

- When have you felt the most grateful and fulfilled?
- Who and what do you love?
- What wild beauty have you not yet unleashed?
- What brings you joy?
- What makes you feel most alive?

As you follow the answers to places where your curiosity is aroused and your energy rises, the expanded self helps you imagine a new agenda, asking: How can you experience more of all that and allow it into this moment? How can you bring this joy, love, gratitude, beauty, and fulfillment—this *life*—into the world now?

Meeting the Wise Self: An Encounter with Beauty

Here is a simple way to evoke and begin to connect with this exuberant adviser, the Wise Self:

Go to a place that moves or delights you, a place that feels sacred to you somehow, and gives you a feeling of coming home. That place may be a spot in nature—a certain seashore or garden, a path along a creek or through the trees—that fills your senses and speaks to your spirit. But you could just as well decide to wander through an art museum and immerse yourself in color. Choose a place that inspires you, puts you in touch with however you define beauty, and leaves you feeling replenished. If your shoulders drop, your lungs expand, and your mind begins to quiet as you enter the space, you're in the right place.

Linger there. Let the rest of the world fall away. If mobility isn't an issue, find a way to walk as you contemplate what's around you, taking both body and mind off their well-beaten paths and allowing them to range into new territory. There's no need to pull out your phone and take photographs for later or check in with someone far away. See what it's like just to be present, looking through the inquisitive, delight-seeking eyes of your Wise Self.

That's it. No homework, no extra-credit assignments. Just identify a place that feels sacred, that uplifts and inspires you. Go there. Fill yourself up. Linger. *Notice* what you're experiencing and savor it. Imagine your Wise Self urging, "Let's do it again." Let that voice begin to edge out the one that might scold, "You don't have time for this." Feel yourself expanding into the beauty around you, coming to life. This is what the Wise Self wants for you.

What Kind of Wisdom Does the Wise Self Possess?

I realize that the joy-seeking Wise Self who revels in beauty may not seem to fit the classic image of the sage, the "profoundly wise person" of the dictionary definition, whom it's easy to imagine as an almost mythic character with flowing white hair and a collection of enigmatic sayings. (I think I'm picturing the "sage on the mountaintop" who's a regular in so many *New Yorker* cartoons.) "I can't pretend to have access to some esoteric truth," my students tell me in so many words. "I wouldn't presume to call myself wise."

But I think you'll see elements of yourself in the most useful definition of wisdom I've found, which comes from my friend and colleague Roger Walsh, a psychiatrist and author. The kind of wisdom he describes in his book *Essential Spirituality* melds emotional, spiritual, and practical intelligence, which gives us the understanding and skill to face the core issues arrayed before us in later life.

To be wise, Walsh says, is to be able to come to terms with the reality that we are small, mortal humans in a seemingly limitless universe. Wisdom, as he sees it, is the ability to find the purpose and meaning in our lives; to make our way in the midst of mystery and uncertainty; to acknowledge our limits; to manage relationships and being alone; and to navigate the suffering, sickness, and death that will eventually come to us all.

By our fifties, sixties, and seventies, we've already begun to tap the inner resources that wisdom requires, and I hope that as you think about Roger Walsh's definition, you can see the wisdom that's already there inside you. Each of your three inner advisers will bring a different kind of intelligence to the process of deepening that wisdom. Death, the keeper of limits, helps us confront time, underlining that it's urgent to come to terms with how we've lived and how we will enter the spiritual territory ahead. The Wise Self can help you recognize your purpose and feel your way toward it using joy, inspiration, and satisfaction as a guide. And the Soul-Centered Adult inside you, whom you'll soon meet, brings practical skills that will help you act on the Wise Self's guidance so you can complete the work that comprises your legacy.

Playful, curious and fluid, the Wise Self insistently steers us from the surface of life into the core, the realm of heart. That interior focus is essential now, as many of the things that we have long turned to for security—jobs, status, the strength of our bodies—begin to ebb. The more we cling to the idea that what's outside us is our primary source of power, happiness, and meaning, the more powerless we feel as those exterior elements diminish or shift in ways we can't control.

But the Wise Self reminds us of the resources inside us that cannot be depleted: Kindness. Equanimity. Gratitude. Forgiveness. Love. We can find our footing and our most meaningful sense of direction and completeness by moving these qualities from the edges of our lives to the center. In doing that, we can root ourselves in what endures through change rather than what will inevitably disappear.

The Third Adviser: The Soul-Centered Adult

Choosing to leave the adult stage and embrace the growth that we're poised to explore in later life doesn't mean forgetting all we know or distancing ourselves from our abilities. We don't stop wanting to create, accomplish, and do. And we don't suddenly lose the adult part of the self that has served our egos so well for so long and helped us achieve so much.

Adult and *ego* aren't husks we have to shed on the journey through our wisdom years. We need them. But now their role shifts. Now, these most capable and dominant parts of ourselves must take a supporting role, stepping aside to make room for the soul's agenda.

It can be a tricky transition because the soul's voice we hear when consulting Death and the Wise Self insists that we take the risk of following impulses and callings we have so far ignored and becoming someone we have not yet been. They are telling us, "There's more to you than your adult habits have allowed you to experience"— and discovering that "more" makes us beginners again, feeling our way along instead of pushing, striving, and striding through our familiar ways of being. We may get lost, stumble, and fall. Or look foolish. Or make many false starts and mistakes. And all of this is uncomfortable to an adult self that prizes achievement, mastery, and acknowledgment. In the name of protecting us, our egos may try to insist that we continue on as before, where it's safe and dignified and "no one will do anything stupid."

It's extremely important, then, to find ways to bring the adult self and ego onboard as valued advisers in this new phase of life, enlisting their support and making clear the key role they have to play now.

I suggest doing this by tapping the adult's natural love for a mission and goals, and asking it to take on the assignment of applying its well-honed abilities to the project of helping you build a soul-centered life.

After consulting Death and the Wise Self, invite the Soul-Centered Adult into the conversation by asking the questions that it's uniquely qualified to help you answer:

- What are you being called to do and be?
- How might you make that happen and give it a life?
- What first steps might you take?
- How would your next ten years look if you committed fully to this direction?
- What would you have to give up to make this happen?
- What would you have to learn?
- Who might best support your new intentions?

The adult self knows all about agency and achievement and is practiced in building structures to support goals and dreams. Now, it has a chance to grow by listening to the voices of the other two advisers. Its role in this time of life is to serve and collaborate rather than command, to realize that you can't bully grace. Sometimes the best action, as the Wise Self can teach, is to wait.

As we all learn, it's not possible to power through the transitions of the wisdom years. While the adult self might well be content to make a list of "the top ten things I want to accomplish in the next ten years" and push you to start crossing them off, such lists will probably look much like extensions of the ones you've made your whole life. Lists alone aren't adequate tools or incentive for re-envisioning your life or breaking decades' worth of habits. What sustains us through the changes of the wisdom years and the process of letting go of what we've been is finding joy in what we might become. Joy, and not will, motivates the adult self to give up its traditional control—and there's nothing more powerful than being thrilled by an alternative view of who you might be and what you might do. Where there's an undercurrent of joy to be tapped, there's an attractive reason for the adult self to pitch in with enthusiasm and set a new course with concrete action. Action is good and necessary—but the Soul-Centered Adult who is emerging now needs to learn that action only serves our growth when it's suffused with the sensibilities of the Wise Self.

Because the adult self is so familiar, I won't go into much more detail here. Knowing that we can rely on its well-honed talents is comforting, and now the trick is to bring a soul focus to the fore. That's something we'll do in coming chapters.

One direct way of creating a new relationship with the adult part of yourself is to consciously consult Death and the Wise Self *before* asking for the adult's input. To ask "What really matters to me?" and "Does it bring me joy?" instead of jumping straight into "What do I need to do?" is a way of resetting routines and allowing the adult self to experience a more soulful and collaborative focus.

Day by day, the adult self will learn to let your Wise Self lead, absorbing Death's messages and, in doing so, it will help you recognize dimensions of personality and existence beyond the ego and explore them.

The Experiment Begins

I can't tell you precisely what will happen as you spend more time with these three advisers and let their sensibilities inform the years ahead. But as you'll see, the more you learn to consult them and, as a result, to experiment with the ideas that begin to bubble up in your consciousness, the more possible it becomes to let old ways of being dissolve and for new possibilities to take their place. You can find out what's yet to be born in you and nurture it into the world.

CHAPTER TWO

THE SECOND TASK

Create Space in your Life for What Wants to Emerge

ppealing as the voice of our Wise Self can be as it prods us to seize any chance to do what makes us happy, we may not know what that is, or be wary of what attracts us. We stall at "What's next?" and "Who do I want to be now?"

Anthropologists tell us that in a traditional culture, we might navigate this transitional time by joining others like us for a rite of passage, a symbolic shedding of the outward trappings of our old life, followed, perhaps, by a period of retreat in which we called to the gods for guidance as we let our old identity dissolve and a new one take shape. Then we might return, transformed and ready for the final phase of our lives.

But our own culture pushes us not to pause and dissolve, feel, and reflect. We're immersed in the paradigm of "successful/active aging," which suggests that our choice is either to speed across the border into later life by staying active as before or to slide into decline. There's little encouragement for staying still long enough to discover who we might be if we set aside the expectations of the past and choose our own goal, our own shape, our own pace, our own course.

"Action" culture is so pervasive that it's almost invisible, and before we can create the space to answer the new callings of later life, it's helpful to understand how staying in a state of constant busyness can crowd out our dreams.

The Problem with "I Need to Stay Productive"

During my "peak performance" years, when I was on the road constantly, speaking and doing consulting work with businesses, I'd often find myself at lunch or dinner with CEOs in their sixties and early seventies who wanted to talk about "what comes next"—how to live a good life after leaving the work that had defined them. They'd say things like "I've been joking that it's going to be all golf and travel for me, but come on. I'd be bored out of my mind. There's only so much time I can spend hitting a little ball around, and how many vacations can you take? My wife talks about seeing the grandkids, who I love, but we can't do that all the time. I feel like sitting at the dock, watching the boats go in and out. Or fishing. It sounds corny, doesn't it? Fishing?"

An admission like that might be followed by an uncomfortable pause and a swing back to talk of work. "I'm thinking of serving on some boards, maybe even starting up a new business . . ." Then they'd get to the crux: "I need to stay productive."

You don't need to come from a business background to be intimately familiar with that thought: *I need to stay productive.* That's what we're supposed to do. That's what gives us worth, we've been told, especially in our later years. We've spent our lives "achieving or producing a significant result" (the dictionary definition of *productivity*) in our jobs and families. And now, if we can just keep it up, we'll age well and hold our value in the world.

That message is all around, from the boardroom to Viagra ads to those ever-popular media features on super-achieving octo- and nonagenarians—a ninety-five-year-old car salesman who just sold his millionth convertible, say, or an eighty-seven-year-old who runs a marathon a month. What's implied in the discussion about "successful aging" is that it's something we can measure externally and strive toward. Maybe we can even get an A.

"Be productive" frequently shares space in our minds with the other imperatives that have pushed us along in life so far: "Stay busy." "Be a success." "Don't let anybody down." "Don't do it if you're not good at it." If we're still working at sixty-eight or seventy, this inner voice says, "Be glad they still want you" and drowns out any sense that we'd rather be doing something else. We may feel like playing with the dogs or pulling down boxes from the garage and rereading old letters. But the adult voice inside won't have it. "If you don't stay busy doing something useful, you'll lose it." "You'll turn into a crumbling, out-of-touch old person."

That voice comes on with so much authority that it's easy to believe it without questioning. But to let your adult self dictate the terms of later life is to miss the possibilities that are just now opening up for you, calling you in new directions. It's as though you're a small child trying to create a vision of yourself as an adolescent when all you have are a child's sensibilities and vocabulary. You love building with Legos now, and maybe you're even known as being something of a Legos master, so why would you want to give that up? When you're older, you imagine, you'll make *bigger* things with Legos, and if you get interested in girls/boys, you'll do Legos together.

"Success" in one form or another has been our "Legos"—the preoccupation that's defined us no matter what activity or mission we've given our days to. We have a difficult time, at first, seeing possibilities that don't revolve around it. But life is much larger and deeper than what fits in a box labeled "success," and in later life we begin to feel an insistent pull toward what lies beyond. It gets harder and harder to keep from wondering: "Is that all there is to me? If there's more, what is it? Who *else* am I besides what I've always done?"

A student of mine, Beth, was an accountant who had always hoped to have a career working with animals but never found a way to make a living doing it. She thought she'd made peace with the way things had turned out and wrote off animal work as an unrealistic fantasy. But when she was in her early sixties, a friend forwarded a quote he'd seen online: "Not everything that counts can be counted. And not everything that can be counted counts." She felt a pang when she read it. What if she'd measured her life on a different scale, she asked herself. What if the love she felt for creatures counted as much as the security and confidence she prized in her job? She knew it wasn't either/or—that she could have both—yet she'd always let the job count for more than most anything else. She pinned the quote above her desk at work and carried on conversations with it. What really counted for her? How would she let herself show it?

This can be uncomfortable territory full of desires, fears, and longings we've long held down. There's a kind of reckoning in which we ask: What have my choices cost me? Have I given up too much? Is it too late to go another way?

It's easy to veer quickly into "doing something productive" instead of waiting for answers or taking the time to nurture the sense that it's legitimate and possible to steer away from what's always brought us security, stability, and respect and find those things in ways that bring fresh satisfaction. Discovery takes patience. We have to give ourselves time to respond to what calls to us, tasting it, trying it on for size, if only in our imaginations. That's why this task of transformation—*create space for what wants to emerge*—is so important.

It's in idle reveries, inklings, and unexpected impulses that we often begin to retrieve forgotten or neglected parts of ourselves, the parts that might have been pushed aside because they didn't fit with the roles we strived to fulfill in adult life: parent, provider, activist, worker, partner, expert, "go-to person who holds things together." Joan Chittister, who writes about aging so beautifully, says that striving isn't really the problem. What's harmful is "the sacrifice of all other dimensions of life in order to achieve it." These sacrificed elements, some familiar, some quite unknown to us, are the keys to our wholeness, the missing pieces of our lives. For my father, who worked as a salesman all his life but longed to go into theater, it was clear that the missing piece was acting, something he pursued with gusto in retirement. But for many of us, it's harder to pin down what's been missing, and it's only when we finally stop trying so hard to succeed and prove ourselves to others that we can sense what has been hovering at the edge of our consciousness.

The feelings, nudges, fantasies, and fascinations that bubble up in moments when you let yourself step away from being "busy" and "productive" are the clues to what's been neglected, what's been waiting for you to remember; they appear in the "nothingness" of silence, stillness, lazy hours, empty slots on the calendar, and daydreaming. This is the open space that is so vital to create for yourself; the realm where it's possible to notice what's gleaming in the corner of your eye, asking for your attention, and to hear your Wise Self asking, "What dream will die in me unless I feed it now?"

Slowing Down Can Be the Kiss of Life

If someone had told me when I was in my late fifties that *idle* time was what would propel me toward the most fulfilling stage of my life, I would've laughed at the irony and said I was way too busy for that. *Ease* was not part of my universe. I didn't make fun of people who talked about relaxation or letting up on the pace or doing things just for the pleasure of it. That was fine for them. But I'd been pushing myself since before kindergarten, and I had no sense of what life would be like if I didn't have to be bigger, better, best, no matter what I took on—not just in the business world, but in my personal life and social service work. In my mind, there was no such thing as stopping; if a goal successfully achieved didn't lead to a more difficult or higher goal, it wasn't worth it. When those questioning CEOs asked what they might do next after their careers, I'm afraid I tacitly discouraged them from the fishing and dreaming they longed for and needed. I didn't say, "Don't do it." I just dismissed their longing reveries by saying, in so many words, "Oh, I could never do that."

I admit I was a hard case. But many of us have our own deeply ingrained sense that there are certain standards we must always reach, a certain kind of focus and strength and competence we *always* have to bring to our lives as leaders or parents or "good examples"—an ability to push on, no matter how tired. That's *who we are.*

Fortunately, for the many of us who spent our adult years feeling driven in one way or another, our bodies eventually begin to tell us that they're not perpetual-motion machines, and our Wise Self finds ways to penetrate the white noise of our nonstop routines to send a quiet message: "I'm done. I can't keep doing this. It's not me anymore." The trick, when this happens, is not to resist or rush past it, but to wander in the place of unknowing where nothing feels quite right anymore. Space opens up around us as we wait for something new to emerge. And quite often, grace flies in through that opening.

I was laid low, at first, during the four years I struggled with my arthritic hip. Because I'd prided myself on being athletic, it was a blow to my ego and my sense of self, not just to my mobility, when suddenly every step I took was slow and painful. Anytime I forgot myself and tried to rush, a stabbing pain brought me back to my new reality: I had to slow down.

I hated knowing that I was now the guy who would still be in the crosswalk when the signal turned, trying to get across. I resented having to sit down so often to rest. I wanted to hike, not be stuck on a park bench. All I could see was diminishment and decline, and as I quietly railed against it, I was a depressed and cranky old man. But as time went on, the slowdown created a kind of spaciousness in me, an unplanned opportunity for reflection. When I sat down to rest, I'd look at the people passing by and wonder about them and how their lives were going. People I'd never noticed—older folks, street people, neighbors walking dogs—began to catch my eye and say hello. I remember being in the middle of a crosswalk when a man slowly going the other way pointed to my hip as I limped by. "Right hip," I said. He pointed to his leg and smiled. "Knee," he said. We both laughed, wounded brothers.

Slowly, almost imperceptibly, a whole world opened up. This steady stream of connection with the people around me was calling to me. I began to enjoy my time in slow motion, the pauses for rest when I'd think about my life, gaze into the trees, pick up ongoing threads of conversation from the day before. All of it, the thinking, the chats, the sense of being woven into my community, receiving small acts of kindness from them and returning smiles and kindness, felt—and feels—as important to me as anything I have ever done. There was so much more to me than my aching hip, so much more to value than the next thing on my list. I felt my reality take shape around the axis of *now*, not some point in the future. And as that happened, I stopped being the guy with better things to do than inhabit his own life. I started to be present there on my corner, on my street, on my bench. I became *intimate* with my life again.

Is this "successful aging"? I'm fairly certain that's not what the success mavens had in mind. But is it rich and satisfying? Yes, it is. It feeds a hunger I never realized I had, and even after surgery replaced my hip and made slowing down less necessary, I'm savoring what I've learned to be.

We have a terribly incomplete model of what it means to grow older. I mentioned the way we tend to celebrate the showy blooms of youth and often feel bereft when the flowers scatter, leaving the branches bare. But I'd like to suggest that what happens next, after the flowers are gone, is the point of it all. The fruit within us ripens invisibly then, the sweet essence of ourselves that we're here to cultivate at this time of life. Our goal now isn't achievement or success for their own sake. It's to tend this fruit—our wisdom, our fascinations, our kindness, our hearts softened by loss and love, selves made sweet and deepened by time—and give it all away.

The slow ripening can start with a subtle nudge toward a calling, a sudden hunger, a new kind of presence, and it draws us ever closer to our core. First, though, we have to make room for the process to happen.

Letting the World Open Up

My friend Harriet, a psychotherapist with a thriving practice, hadn't given any thought to slowing down. She planned to keep going full steam ahead "forever," and she had enough energy at seventy to make that seem like a real possibility. She had been seeing clients back to back, forty hours a week, for almost four decades, and she had always taken pride in helping people through their life crises and seeing them gain insight into themselves. She was thankful to be in a profession where experience and wisdom count, and where she could feel as though she was in her prime at her age, only getting better.

So she was startled when she heard a client in the middle of a session obviously trying to get her attention. "I thought I was listening," she told me, "but my mind had wandered off. It was so embarrassing, and so unlike me." She spent the next months paying close attention to what she was experiencing during her work hours and realized that something had shifted for her. "So often I'd just feel impatient with all those people and their problems," she said. "I'd look out the window and want to get outside. I think I'd been on autopilot for a while, but now it was obvious to me."

Shifting into autopilot is common as we reach the end of our old path. At the very time when an inner urgency is building for change, we're often knowingly or unknowingly withdrawing energy from what we've always done.

Harriet decided to cut back her hours and work part-time, giving herself the option of filling her schedule again after she "recharged." "I couldn't in good conscience work with my full roster of clients if I couldn't be present with them when they needed me," she said. Her plan was to use her freed-up time to work on a book that described her approach to therapy, something she could share with both clients and other therapists.

The prospect of having so many open slots on her calendar made her nervous, though, and she quickly filled them up. She volunteered to set up a counseling program at her church and devoted more volunteer hours to a counseling program for teens, on top of seeing clients and blocking out four hours a day for writing her book. She laughed when I told her it sounded as though she hadn't cut back on working at all and, indeed, was working more than ever. "It's true," she said. "I was almost afraid to be alone with myself."

But Harriet chafed against the new schedule she'd put in place, especially the writing. She'd sit down to think about her book and almost immediately feel tired or distracted. "I really battled myself," she said. "I was determined to do what I said I was going to do. But I was so relieved when the gardener would come. I'd have an excuse to get out of my chair and go watch him with the plants. It made me happy to get out of my head and wade into all that beautiful color. I could feel myself relax."

After a month or two of that, she started asking the gardener to show her how she could help out with the flower beds. "Not just the fun stuff like planting and cutting blooms to bring inside," she told me, "but trimming back the dead stalks and pulling weeds. I like the physical work of it, the way my mind gets quiet. I can't explain it, but I love seeing that world up close, the whole life cycle, beginning to end. You know the great thing? Plants don't need a therapist," she added with a laugh. "They respond to the care you give them, but they have their own kind of knowing about what comes next. They don't want my advice. Just my care."

My sense, and hers too, is that there's much more going on in the garden for her than tending the dahlias and poppies. Because she's let herself give in to its persistent, delicious call, the world has grown larger than her treatment room, larger than a series of problems to be solved, and her mind and heart are wandering into it. She isn't trying to analyze the experience. She's immersing herself in it.

Gardening wasn't part of Harriet's careful plan for her life, but it's become the part of her day she most looks forward to—and she's stopped rushing back to something "more pressing." Digging in the dirt felt incidental to her at the beginning, a way of procrastinating from the work she was supposed to be doing, the people she was supposed to help. But it's become central to her. It makes her feel alive.

That's the clue to the rightness of whatever calls or intrigues you as you make time for discovery: the feeling of aliveness it sparks in you. I'm not suggesting that you do what I did or make Harriet your model. I have no prescription for you that says, "Go sit on a park bench," or "Find your way in later life by gardening!" Whatever gestures in your direction and feels meaningful to you will be highly personal. *Meaningful* is something only you can define. It may seem eccentric, irrational, or like a waste of time to someone else. But the cookie cutter part of life is over. You're free to listen for and pursue your intuitions— the life you are culminating, enriching, and ripening is yours and no one else's. There's no competition, nothing to prove. Your sense of aliveness is enough. *You* are enough.

You may not believe that yet. But what would you do if it were true?

"But What if What I Want to Do Is Watch YouTube Videos?"

I know it can be hard to let "Do whatever calls you" feel like an acceptable choice if you've always prioritized doing your duty and being good at what you do. So I want to share one more story of what it can look like to set out in a direction that may seem hard to justify to the part of yourself that's still telling you to "Be productive."

Larry had had a long and successful career as an investment banker but started feeling restless when he was in late fifties. "I was making a lot of money—too much to want to quit—but I realized I just didn't have the same intensity I used to," he told me. "I was tired, a little bored. It was way too early to think about retiring, and I'd sit in my office or on my commute home wondering what my problem was.

"I've given my family a good life, but it kind of bothered me that my kids had no idea, really, of what I do. My whole life came down to numbers on a page. Whatever I was going to leave them was numbers on a page. I thought about this a lot when my old man got sick. He worked with his hands all his life—he built things. I always wanted to.

"Around that time, I had a memory of being a kid and watching this woodworking show on Saturday mornings. A guy cutting up wood and nailing it together, basically. I couldn't get enough of it. I wondered if they still had stuff like that on TV, so I went on YouTube. I couldn't find the exact show, but there was a whole *world* of videos on carpentry."

Larry plunged in. It gave him such escapist pleasure to watch guys turning piles of lumber into walls and wainscoting that he started clicking away to the videos when he needed a break from work or in the evening when he'd otherwise have been answering email. "I liked thinking about the process of making things, seeing how somebody did it," he said. He'd once planned to become a civil engineer, but in college someone had noticed his high marks in advanced math and recruited him to work in a financial firm. He never looked back and had no nostalgia for the path he hadn't taken. But there it was when he started watching the woodworking videos—that old fascination with building things.

His YouTube time wasn't something he discussed with anyone. It felt like a dorky, guilty pleasure. He watched because it was better than working, and often that time became a portal into his thoughts. He mused about his dad, a man who'd spent his life as a laborer. His mind skipped through his past. Larry wasn't watching porn or playing video poker, he told himself, so he let it be okay to hang out with the carpenters building cabinets and hand-turning table legs on the screen. It looked like fun and reminded him of how much he had loved the handcrafted furniture he'd been surrounded with growing up. That was something he thought he'd outgrown years ago when he moved into a minimal, modern house.

As he thought and watched and remembered, Larry didn't suddenly quit his job or make a drastic change. He continued on as before, but let himself drift into reveries, sometimes watching the videos closely and becoming interested in the process he was seeing, sometimes daydreaming and lingering in the quiet afterward. He began remembering what he liked, what *he* was like. That's another way this fertile "fallowness" can feel—like meandering in a world within a world, a time out of regular time when simply being who you are, enjoying what you enjoy, is more important than busily doing what you're supposed to.

Finding the Sacred Spaces of Your Life

In the borderlands between the endings of adulthood and the new beginnings of later life, there's a chance to sink into ourselves, revisiting where we've been, looking with new eyes at what's around and within us. What we're searching for finds us in our slowing and stillness and silence. These are the wellsprings of intimacy with ourselves, the world, and the divine, and they become central, fittingly, at the time of our lives when our bodies and spirits are often asking us to learn to treat them more gently, to learn patience, to stop pushing so hard, and give in to what we'd most like to do.

Harriet, Larry, and I stumbled into this transition unprepared, but I encourage you to make an *intentional* practice of easing yourself into a kind of quiet receptiveness where you can hear your own inner promptings. An excellent and deeply satisfying way to do that is to find and spend time in your own sacred spaces—places that your body responds to with a feeling of calm and "coming home": a rose garden, a spot in the park, a seashore, or a hill with a view of a sparkling night sky. There, you can fill your senses, connect to what expands beyond you and inside you. I'm lucky enough to live not far from redwood forests that fill me with awe, but your sacred space might be the corner where you like to watch the sky coloring at sunset or a particular corner of your yard where the burbling of a fountain gives you a sense of peace. Harriet's garden is certainly a sacred space for her—you don't have to travel a great distance to travel far.

Perhaps even more important is creating a sacred space for yourself in your home, and a sacred time that is all your own, clear of the outside world and exterior demands, free of news, the internet, and other people's thoughts. This sanctuary—whether it's a private study or office or a chair at the kitchen table in the early morning quiet when you can be alone—is made sacred by your regular attention, your listening, your patience. All that's required is your willingness to keep returning.

What will you do in your sacred place and time? Anything that calls you into yourself and your own thoughts and desires rather than bouncing you into the always-running world.

You may want to create a simple ritual that begins and ends your sacred time and marks it as sacred. Simply lighting a candle when you begin and blowing it out when you "leave" can be a signal that this time is yours for the purpose of communing with yourself and stands apart from the rest of the day or night. One of my friends settles into a comfortable chair with a hot drink first thing in the morning, takes three slow, deep breaths, and inwardly says, "I'm back," to mark the beginning of her sacred time. Then she sits with her journal and writes down her dreams, thinks her thoughts. When she's finished she purposely stops for another three deep breaths to bring the time to a close. Another person I know puts on music that moves him and sits immersed in it, letting his mind wander.

I meditate in my sacred space, the room where I do much of my thinking and creative work. Some people pray or paint or knit. I think it's helpful to think of your sacred time as a chance to become reacquainted with a good friend you haven't seen in a while, meeting that person with intimate curiosity, letting silence and activity come as they come. Will you always feel like sitting and reflecting? Probably not. You may decide to take a walk, pull a book off the shelf and page through it, bring in a cutting from the garden, drag a chair to the window and watch it snow. But in all that, keep circling back to yourself, remaining outside ordinary time and its endless demands.

As you work with this book, you might carry its questions and exercises into your sacred time. Ask "What has meaning for me now?" or "What would I love to do next?" and see where your mind and heart and inspirations take you.

If you find that after just a few minutes your mind has sped ahead to bills and work and appointments and all the activities of the day, it can be helpful to use a simple, meditative practice to ground yourself.

Nothing exotic; just breathing. You can shift your state and slow your thoughts with deep, even breaths. Inhale slowly through your nose, then count *one* on the first slow exhale. Let the exhale be even longer than the inhale. Count *two* on the second exhale, three on the third, all the way to ten.

Or peel an orange, mindfully and with care, noticing and appreciating the layers of sensation that flow from such an ordinary act. Feel the weight of the globe in your palm, and then watch the fine mist of scented oil that sprays as you pierce the skin and peel a strip away. Notice the contrast between the bright orange of the surface and the smooth, white pith inside.

As you breathe in the sharp, sweet scent of orange, you might detect traces of the orange tree's candy-sweet blossoms or remember the fruit tucked into your lunchbox many years ago or think of an old lover's perfume. When the process of peeling and sensing carries you all the way to the juicy prize inside, pull out one segment, then bite into it, savoring the taste. You're here, awake, connected to what's available to you when you slow down the world.

Gently tuning into your senses, your breathing, and your thoughts, brings you back into company with yourself, listening, observing, paying attention to your life, and how it feels to you now. What's bringing you pleasure? What's coming to an end? What has juice for you?

Sacred comes from a root word meaning *holy*—dedicated to God or, in a related sense, to *wholeness*. Creating this sacred space and time is a way of calling in the parts of yourself that have been scattered and overshadowed. What makes you feel *whole* now?

In slowing to ask and notice what we're feeling and sensing, we open ourselves to the unexpected richness of our lives, waking to the beauty that only emerges when we are there to see. As the late Irish priest and poet John O'Donohue tells us, "Beauty waits until the patience and depth of a gaze are refined enough to engage and discover it." I think that's true not only of the beauty in the world around us, but of the beauty in other people—and in the parts of ourselves we've yet to unfurl.

By the time we reach later life, we're extremely accomplished at doing. But we're often much less practiced at being present with our lives, and it's crucial to learn how. It's not that later life is devoid of action and accomplishment—far from it. But without cultivating this time of waiting, listening, and reorienting ourselves around what brings us to life, it's easy to be driven by old habits, old fears. Begin to transform yourself by creating space and silence that allow you to give priority to what longs to bloom. Open yourself to what brings you joy.

CHAPTER THREE

THE THIRD TASK

Gravitate toward Joy

I t's common to stumble into unexpected storehouses of joy as you reset your inner compass and become ever more sensitive to the call of new fascinations, long-buried interests, and forgotten or neglected loves and dreams. That's what we've been doing so far, in this transition zone between adulthood and later life: shifting our sense of true north from the exterior pull of duty to the much deeper callings of the heart.

There's a powerful pleasure that comes with feeling your way toward your own desires and claiming a life that you've cut precisely to your own shape, and that pleasure draws you into the territory of the Wise Self. It opens the door for wisdom itself.

It can be challenging at first to proceed this way, turning inward for guidance and working to find the courage to seek no one's permission but your own to steer toward whatever beckons. But building those capacities, gravitating toward joy, begets the play, fulfillment, flow, and sense of expansion that are available to you in the wisdom years. Joy is the signal that a direction you're considering is right for you, and it urges you to continue on that way.

When I talk about joy, I don't mean bubbly, giggly, too-much-champagne euphoria or the rush of winning the lottery, though there's nothing wrong with those. I'm thinking instead about an inner fire that sparkles in the eyes, a fire that sometimes flares into exuberance and bliss and sometimes takes the form of a quiet glow of gratitude, pleasure, or contentment.

Researchers who study the emotions have identified scores of varieties of joy, and you'll see many definitions that try to capture its essence, but for the purposes of this book, I'd like to describe it this way:

Joy is the sense of happiness and well-being that comes from connecting deeply with what makes us feel most alive.

It doesn't require money, extraordinary good luck, or even circumstances that seem positive to cultivate joy. But because joy is born of nurturing our connection to what genuinely has meaning for us, what *lights us up*, finding it does require paying attention to what produces those inner sparks and experimenting to discover what else might.

I can't tell you exactly what will allow you to commune with joy—finding out, after all, is a highly personal mission. But I *can* tell you how you'll recognize it: When you engage with something that brings you joy, time disappears and you're immersed in the experience, absorbed. The exchange, however brief or long, enlarges you, moves you, kindles you. And in response, joy flows into your heart, then back to the world.

Joy happens in the present. It's possible only when "Be here now" replaces "Be there then." It's a feeling, not a competition; so there's no trophy attached, no need to climb a peak, no rating system, no gold star for trying harder. There's no goal attached, no requirement that there be some sort of growth involved or any sort of peak experience.

All it requires is giving yourself over to what holds the most meaning and delight for you, an endlessly varied list that might include making something with your hands, walking with a friend, swooning over a book, playing with a beloved animal companion, feeling a grandchild snuggle up for a story, or losing yourself in art or nature.

I hope you've already begun opening the door to what delights you because the more you allow yourself to do that, the more awake and alive you become; time expands around you, along with the infectious pleasure that comes from letting your life fill up with reflections and expressions of your genuine self. Joy can become the filter through which you see what the world presents to you and what you can offer back. It's a balm for sadness and a light that always draws us back to ourselves and this moment, which is deeper with possibilities than we know.

Joy May Not Be Where You Think
(But You'll Find It by Paying Attention to What You *Feel*)

Most people I know didn't plan for later life by asking: "What would bring me joy?" and listening inward to find it. We often have an idea of what we'd like to do—travel, volunteer, read more books, spend time with family—and sometimes we create fairly detailed plans for projects or bucket-list adventures. But those itineraries may have been drawn up by an adult self whose underlying assumption was that life is a never-ending self-improvement project, with extra points for good works, security, respectability, and "fun photos on Facebook." Such plans sometimes lean heavily on the limited repertoire of "What you're supposed to do when you retire/the kids leave home/you're sixty-five" and "What all my friends are doing." They often come from the head, not the heart.

That was true for Larry, the financial analyst who became so fascinated with woodworking videos. As he got closer to retiring, he couldn't see himself spending all day at home "Playing at some hobby," he told me, so he looked into volunteering with a nonprofit, which could never have afforded his kind of expertise otherwise.

He realized he'd been self-absorbed while he was working and thought volunteering would be a way to remedy that. He liked the idea of becoming an "executive mentor," and his wife had been enthusiastic to hear that he had some sort of plan for the months that stretched ahead. "But as it turned out, it wasn't for me," he said. He enjoyed meeting the nonprofit's staff and quickly saw how he could help, but he soon found that he dreaded seeing his appointments with them on his calendar. "It was the same old same old—numbers and money," he said, and he found it exhausting. He stuck with it as long as he could, but finally, he made up an excuse and got out of the commitment, feeling dissatisfied and a little ashamed, as though he'd somehow "failed" volunteering.

Actually, it took guts to quit. I've seen many people stick with joyless volunteer jobs because they think they must. Often, they've been so defined by their adult careers and roles and have so much invested in them, that on a deep level they believe that "the role is who I am, and the absence of it is the absence of me." When that's the case, losing a title, a set of important responsibilities, or a predictable routine—even one that lost its appeal long ago—can feel like a death, and a volunteer position can offer a semblance of a replacement, filling a hole on the calendar and providing a ready-made sense of purpose.

It's often quite simple to recreate a new life that looks a lot like what came before, sans paycheck. But when I meet people who describe their post-career activities with statements like "At least it gets me out of the house," I often wonder what *calling* they might be ignoring.

"Callings" are sometimes taken to be grand missions etched on us at birth and single-mindedly followed for life or strokes of passion revealed in a lightning flash—both of which make a lot of people think they don't have them. But our callings, I believe, are quite different than that. They're prompts from our deepest being, our joy. What's calling to us is our own profound need to be who we are and offer back to life the gifts that flow from our nature. Turning away from our inner promptings—which often evolve over time, pointing us to layers of ourselves that want expression—leaves a devastating absence in our lives: the absence of our *self*. And that's a hole much larger than a gap in the calendar.

So it's heartening to see that when we're caught in a life that feels dull or deadening, any small joy can begin to call us home.

For Larry, carpentry had been a private fantasy, an almost secret joy, but his derailed experiment with volunteering seemed to provide the excuse he needed to go deeper. "I thought, *What the hell. I flunked volunteering, so I've got time. I'll borrow a few tools and see what happens.* He told me he hesitated initially and considered jumping back into mentoring at another nonprofit but, almost as soon as the thought came to mind, he realized that he wanted a break from his past so he could try something entirely new.

Though Larry by now had probably watched enough videos to have built and furnished an entire house in his imagination, he had to face the enormous gulf between his skills and the ones he'd admired on YouTube when he tried to recreate simple projects in his garage. His first attempts were primitive, as you might expect. But he liked the weight of the hammer and the way it felt to be grappling with materials. He was fascinated with the idea that he might learn to shape something solid and lasting—maybe even beautiful—with his own hands. He committed to kitting out a workshop, with the idea that he'd teach himself to make simple furniture.

From the beginning, everything from the smell of sawdust to his clumsy attempts to match up mitered corners has given him a kind of delight that had long been missing from his life. The game of it, the way everything else disappears as he creates his puzzle pieces and fits them together, absorbs him, even when the results don't seem to reflect the effort he's put in. He enjoys the trial and error and the process of figuring things out, seeking out people who can help him when he gets stuck. His sons, he told me, have taken to dropping by the garage to talk, something he thought would never happen. He's having fun flexing this part of himself. It's impossible to miss his joy.

When Service Truly Calls

I want to spend a little time talking about the idea of service as a source of joy because I know that for many of us the call that comes from the heart pulls us directly toward serving others, be they humans or animals or trees. It can happen when you're walking down the street and feel drawn to respond to a homeless person or when you hear about an organization that's working to solve a problem that's deeply significant to you.

When that's the case, volunteering or otherwise offering yourself to others can be as right for you as it was wrong for Larry when he tried the first time.

I've seen and vividly experienced the joy that comes when people share their talents and their *being* with those who need them. At Shanti, the organization I founded to offer companionship and care to people at the end of life, I've watched many later-life volunteers discover the thrill and gratification that can come from easing the suffering of another person. I've also seen how much connection, pleasure, and purpose can flow from working with others to serve the greater good.

Just as neglected or abandoned parts of ourselves beckon in later life, so do our higher values—compassion, kindness, service—as we begin to ask how we're meant to share our gifts with the world. In later life, we increasingly wonder if what we did mattered, if our time here has made a difference, and it's often liberating to realize that regardless of what has defined us until now, we can still bring our sense of "what really matters" to the center of our lives. This isn't an intellectual decision; it's a matter of the heart. And its hallmark is joy. Thus, even though my end-of-life work and the far-flung volunteer communities it has created have brought me tremendous fulfillment, and I can recommend this work as beautiful and life-changing, I would also say this: in service work, be guided by your *own* feeling of joy. Not mine. What satisfies, uplifts, and produces joy in me might be a grind or an obligation to you. In which case, keep feeling for a better match.

For a writer friend, the right match has been teaching a weekly drop-in writing workshop for homeless people at a local community center. She comes home from her time there feeling moved, connected to her students, and inspired by their work. Giving her time to them produces more in her to give—that's the nature of activities that bring us joy. They refill us. Another friend, who had been weighed down by the sadness of never having children, has become a Big Brother to a boy who's introduced him to Fidget Spinners, the challenges of today's elementary school homework, and the excitement of seeing a shy little boy flourish under his loving attention.

There are countless ways to be of service in every part of our lives, ways to put ourselves in the path of grace and to experience joy in one of the best ways possible—by sharing it. But I know how easy it can be to say, "I ought to volunteer," and create another time-filling obligation that holds no genuine meaning for you. At Shanti, I want the volunteers to find purpose with the mission of our organization and feel the joy of being part of something much larger than their own lives. I want them to feel excited as they see how the compassion they give others produces so much more aliveness in both the clients and themselves. At the same time, I want them to create and be and do the things they've left undone or unexpressed in their own homes, families, hearts, and selves—and not make their service with us a replacement for that.

If volunteering with us does not spark genuine, heart-filling joy, then I hope they'll search for what does. And I wish the same for you, in whatever service role you may consider.

Experiments in Joy
What is it that draws *you* in? What beckons to be discovered or explored? If you've made the effort to slow the pace of your life a bit and notice what flits into your daydreams and Google searches, you may have a notion or two of what interests are stirring. What's taking shape in your imagination? What possibilities feel exciting to you?

If you're game to leap into joy, think about the question I often pose in workshops: What sorts of activities would *thrill* you?

You may have a clear vision, or no clarity at all, but as answers to that enticing question come to mind—some of which you may quickly discount as unrealistic fantasies or "selfish indulgences"—I propose experimenting with them, trying them out the way you might have as an adolescent, when you learned to "adult" by adventuring, testing, tasting what looked appealing and venturing into territory that may have seemed risky or even forbidden.

It often happens that what feels the riskiest and most compelling, at this time of life, has to do with what we've left unexplored. For people who have been consumed with work at the expense of their families, it can feel risky to admit that they're hungry to get to know their adult children again and spend time with their grandchildren. For those who've held in their wildness to "set a good example," the most satisfying risks might come in letting a freak flag fly.

Our culture offers tremendous support for the explorations of youth and understands that period of life as a time of testing things out. But it but has no sense of older people doing that, even though later life can be a period of radical self-discovery. Any experiments we do now may be labeled "desperate" by those who expected us to quietly continue on as before. "Now that you have nothing significant to do, maybe you could take more vacations," the voices around us say. (Yes, they can be quite dismissive!)

But the experiments we try now and the larger changes they set in motion can be as powerful and profound as the ones we tried when we were dreaming up our adult selves as teenagers. As we pivot toward joy, new possibilities begin to excite us, refueling us for this leg of the journey.

Giving Ourselves Permission to Experience Joy

What stops us from eagerly exploring what we want to be now? Sometimes, as in Larry's case, we don't consider orienting our lives around a new source of joy because that would carry us away from our familiar script and fall outside our definition of who we are. We may not have the sort of mental grammar that lets us put "woodworker" in the same sentence that began with "financial analyst" or let "novelist" follow "accountant" and easily allow our identity to shift.

But sometimes—often, even—the resistance has its roots in a fear of upsetting someone, living or dead, who might not approve.

If you look back at the definition of joy, the words "connecting deeply with what makes us feel most alive" aren't followed by any qualifiers about how doing this joyful thing isn't really joy unless it pleases someone else or makes us look good. Yet we often have the idea that it's not worth doing something unless we can do it well or can earn someone's enthusiastic notice and praise. You may have depended on others' approval as a child or used people's admiration as a measure of success as you climbed through the adult world, but the wisdom years insist that *you* are the author of your own life. It's time, says the Wise Self, to offer yourself your *own* approval and to reanimate sources of joy that were shut off long ago because someone suggested it would be better that way.

I hope you'll pause to take this in: *You have the power to pursue your own joy.*

I get a daily demonstration of the freedom that's unleashed when we claim that power from my wife, Cindy Spring, who has a morning ritual of cranking up show tunes, getting on the elliptical, and pouring every bit of her energy into exuberantly singing along. I know that sounds like a perfectly ordinary activity, but for many years, Cindy didn't let herself do it, and her decision to unleash her voice now has been liberating.

She first got the idea that she wanted to sing as she swooned over Elvis Presley in the 1950s. Stirred and inspired, she covered the walls of her room with posters of the King, and when she was twelve years old, she asked her parents for singing lessons. As she tells the story:

"We found a teacher a couple of miles away. Mr. Rudy worked out of a music shop—a long and narrow store filled with dusty musical instruments for sale or rent. I had to walk past the guitars and saxophones to get to the back room where he had an upright piano and lots of sheet music. I remember that he looked a bit like Captain Kangaroo, with a friendly handlebar mustache."

Cindy was a devoted student, going for weekly lessons, then holing up in her room to practice scales and songs. She delighted in finding her voice, confident of her progress.

"Just before the holidays, Mr. Rudy said I should work on 'White Christmas' by Irving Berlin. I practiced and practiced," she remembers, "and I proudly belted it out at my next lesson."

And then the unthinkable happened.

"When I finished, I remember distinctly how Mr. Rudy took his hands off the piano keys and swiveled his chair around toward me. Kindly and clearly he said, 'I think you should think about a different hobby.'"

Cindy was devastated. "It was one of my first failures in life," she says, and while she often made light of it, the wound was deep and lasting. She stopped singing except when she was alone. (It didn't help that a jazz musician boyfriend along the way asked her not to sing when he was in the house.) The Mr. Rudy story became an anecdote she often shared as an adult, one in which Mr. Rudy eventually became a hero for saving her from a mediocre life of chasing a singing career in smoky lounges. The sting faded. But she kept her early passion locked away, and I hardly ever heard her sing.

Then, when she was in her early sixties, we got tickets for a one-man show in which the actor and musician Hershey Felder played

Irving Berlin. Felder recounted Berlin's life story and played dozens of his greatest hits on a grand piano.

Near the end of the show, he asked the audience to stand and sing "White Christmas" while he played the piano. I expected Cindy to silently mouth the words, or keep her voice down, as she usually did. But this time, something swung open in her. "In a room of several hundred people, I let myself belt out the old tune," she remembers. "I had tears running down my face. I couldn't hold back the part of me that loved to sing, and the joy that singing gave me. This time I wasn't going to be quiet."

When we got home, she asked me to sit down in the living room and told me, "I need to sing again, when and where I feel like it. I know I can't carry a tune or stay in key, but something in me has always wanted to sing."

She's been doing it with gusto ever since.

I often stick my head through the door as I'm passing by just so I can see her joyful face as she sings along with "My Fair Lady."

I share that story at length because I think many of us have Mr. Rudys in our lives and assume that the way to push beyond their judgments is to prove them wrong by succeeding where they thought we would fail. But there was no need for Cindy to take singing lessons again, perfect her voice, and show up Mr. Rudy by winning a contest with her moving rendition of "White Christmas." All she had to do was let herself sing, her way, just for the love of it.

The prize is the feeling of rightness and comfort in her own skin that she nurtures as she sings, and the full-body pleasure of that daily gift of joy.

EXERCISE:

Reclaim the Silenced Parts of Yourself

You may not need to reclaim your voice in the literal way Cindy did. But there may be parts of yourself that have been silenced in response to an inner or outer critic or skeptic.

- Are there any onetime joys that you've pushed aside because someone laughed?
- In the name of experimenting with joy, what abandoned fascinations might you revisit?
- What stories do you tell about past failed attempts or embarrassments that might hold clues to interests that you might sample once more?

One friend has often told the story of how her attempts to bake bread back in college in the seventies consistently produced "the most delicious-smelling whole-wheat bricks" she's ever seen. She loved the kneading and pounding, the smells, the textures, the whole experience. "Unfortunately for me, I just don't have that baker's touch," the story typically concludes. She laughs, but I can always detect a twinge of regret.

What might happen now, I wonder, if she circled back to see if the pleasure is still there? This time around, there would be a wealth of new recipes and step-by-step videos to walk her through. Or it could be that she'd find related pleasures working with clay.

As you call to mind old pleasures and "failed attempts," look closely at the elements that made you happiest. Lining them up and imagining ways to remix them in other activities might also lead you toward joy.

The goal here isn't to find a new hobby. It's much larger than that. Allowing yourself to seek and reconnect with what absorbs and compels and delights you is a way of declaring ownership of what was lost, and your intention to reclaim it so you can move through this period of life feeling whole, with more delight to give.

Shifting Your Eyes from the Goal to the Moment

What people sometimes misunderstand about joy is that it's not focused on a result. It flows from the *process* of being connected to what's meaningful to us. As the Buddha is said to have commented, "There is no path to happiness. Happiness is the path." But it can be surprisingly hard to shake the idea that "If I do this thing and accomplish this goal, or improve myself in a particular way, *then* I will be joyful."

An acquaintance of mine, Marion, learned this in a beautiful way not long ago. When she phased out a long career as an office manager in her sixties, she decided that she wanted to cultivate her spiritual life. An idea that caught her imagination was that she might "jump-start" the process by making a pilgrimage to the Camino de Santiago. The Camino, a network of roads and trails that crosses hundreds of miles in France, Spain, and Portugal, culminates at the tomb of St. James in northwest Spain.

Marion hoped that a days-long walk on a literal spiritual path, surrounded by religious pilgrims, might open her to the sort of spiritual awakening that could come from emptying her mind, putting many miles on a pair of shoes, and committing herself to the sacred. "I didn't want a vacation," she said. "I wanted something meaningful, and I think that underneath everything, I wanted a huge jolt of transformation that would push me into a truly committed spiritual life. Like Paul on the road to Damascus."

She spent weeks plotting out the trip and thinking about the holiness, or at least wholeness, that might rise from the dust and somehow change her.

But the sense of joy she'd thought would repay her effort didn't come. Her travels had been . . . interesting, she told me. She had stories to tell, and she was glad she went. But there was no great glow of satisfaction, no lightning bolt of conversion or enlightenment. Just a sense of "Huh. I guess that wasn't it."

Restless when she got home, she took herself to the Asian Art Museum in San Francisco, which has long been one of her favorite places. She's always loved to circle through the new exhibitions, and she returns again and again to the pieces she loves most, transported by their colors and stories and company. The galleries are her turf, her home ground.

Marion never studied art history or tried to make art herself, but she's always felt she was stepping into a larger world in the presence of fine art, an experience that she has mostly kept private, not trying to put into words what she feels as she lingers in front of a painting or sculpture others might glance at without really seeing. She's used to being the one who has to be told when it's closing time.

When the plan to "come home transformed" fell apart, she began spending more time walking and thinking at the museum, and on one of those trips she talked with a docent, who noticed her enthusiasm and suggested she might become a docent herself.

Marion jumped at the idea.

"My soul comes alive in the museum," she told me. Recognizing that has allowed her to make joy an active part of her daily life. She didn't have to earn it with a pilgrimage or adopt a new religion or look for outside intervention; it wasn't a prize at the end of the path. Her "road to Damascus" was in front of her and inside her, familiar and beloved.

EXERCISE:

Return to Reliable Sources of Joy

As you think about where your joy may lie, consider the places, people, and activities you're drawn to, the ones that reliably elevate your spirit. What always gives you a sense of hope, inspiration, or uplift? What makes you feel like yourself again? Where do you go and what do you do to replenish yourself when you feel depleted?

List them.

How could you bring more of *that* into your life? What might you do in the next week to experience it?

"At *My* Age?"

Connecting with the joy that comes with doing something just for the love of it may require finding the courage to keep going against expectations or assumptions about what's possible, "reasonable," or "acceptable." Almost any time in life, it can feel precarious to step into the unknown, drawn by a desire that may not yet make sense to anyone else. But that feeling can be compounded by the words "At my age?"

One remedy for the doubts and resistance, I've found, is to remind ourselves of the life-altering and affirming times when we've made the choice to follow our own light. Let me suggest a simple exercise we do in my workshops:

EXERCISE:

When Did You Take a Chance on Yourself?

Remember a time when you took the risk of breaking from the status quo in your life to go your own way. Visualize where you were and who surrounded you. What inspired you to make the change? Did you consider it for a long time or was it sudden? What happened as a result? What surprised you?

These breaks from the expected can lead to some of the most charged and meaningful experiences of our lives, the times when we took a chance on our own instincts. Was this such a time for you? How did the experience change you?

When I put these questions to a workshop recently, one man, Frank, was quick to answer. Earlier in the session he had made a couple of mentions of how he'd taken a year off at age twenty-five to travel around the world and animatedly described the adventures he'd had hitchhiking and camping out. The trip clearly stood as a high point almost fifty years later. Telling us of what he'd learned then, he said, "People want the same things everywhere. They want to be happy, they want to nurture their families, and they want to be proud of themselves."

What he added to the story now were details about how that experience had changed the direction of his life when he returned. At first, the apparent answer was "not at all." As soon as he'd hung up his hiking boots, he took a corporate job, rising to a senior position in a real estate firm. The money was great, Frank said, but he was burned out by forty. So he decided to take a break to renew himself. Once again he hit the road as a wanderer with no set destination. But this time, when his trip was over, he shocked himself and everyone in his life by quitting his job and training to become a social sciences teacher.

That was the risk he told our group about: giving up the money and security of his real estate job to share his love of geography and world culture with high school and then junior college students. "It was the risk that made all the difference in my life," he said, beaming. He'd been a blissful teacher.

As he got into his seventies, though, all that courage and adventure seemed far in the past. When I asked him what he was most excited about doing in his wisdom years, his face clouded. "I'm not sure," he said.

"Let me go out on a limb and ask if you've thought about traveling," I said.

He gave me an irritated look. "You know what it takes to take that kind of big trip?" he asked. "I'd love to do it, but I'm not twenty-five, or even forty anymore."

"How about a tour?"

"A tour? On a bus with a bunch of old people?"

The group laughed.

"Maybe not the kind of tour you think," I said. "There are tours for older people that focus on just what you're interested in, going to 'real' places, interacting with people, sticking around long enough to get an immersive feel for the culture." I mentioned that he might want to check out the "elderhostel" concept, now called "Road Scholar," whose name is a tip-off to its more serious intent.

Frank was pulling out his phone to Google "Road Scholar" almost before we finished talking.

Why hadn't he thought about this fairly obvious option before? I think the reason many of us don't see the possibility of revisiting the joys of the past is that we associate them with our youth, not our nature, and mistakenly believe that when youth is gone—whether it's our twenties or our forties—so is the joy, not realizing that we can still find that feeling of deep connection with what we love.

We can be surprisingly literal in the "requirements" we ascribe to joy. Frank had unconsciously assumed that because he couldn't do exactly the same sort of trip he'd taken at twenty-five, he couldn't have a "genuine" experience of travel. But as our group members pointed out, "You're not supposed to redo that trip, and you wouldn't want to. You're not the same person you were." Perhaps, setting out now, he'd seek out different, deeper conversations; companions with long life experience to share; a slower pace with more time to absorb what he was seeing. In doing that, he'd take a risk equal to his earlier ones as he let himself break through the idea that the transformations of travel and cultural connection are available only to the young.

The Joy Filter

You can invite joy into your life by embracing something that fills you with a sense of enduring pleasure and deep satisfaction, as many of the people in this chapter have done. But you can also do it by ceasing a part of your life that has outlived its capacity for triggering joy, if it ever had one. That might involve ending a duty-filled career, handing off a set of obligations that have weighed you down, or dissolving a relationship that's always been based on practicalities instead of love. But the shift you make needn't be dramatic. You might find great joy in simply doing more of what you love and less of what you don't.

A while back, a book on "tidying up" the home by Japanese author Marie Kondo, soared to the top of the best-seller lists. Her core technique for sorting through clutter and creating serene, well-ordered spaces was to ask of each item in a closet, drawer or room: "Does it spark joy?"

People reported filling huge trash bags, trucks, and dumpsters with joyless discards, and Kondo provided careful instructions for folding, arranging, and honoring what was left.

"Does it spark joy?" is a question the Wise Self loves, and I highly recommend it as a filter for looking anew at what fills your calendar now, deciding what deserves space, time, and a place of honor. Sitting with your datebook and reviewing your commitments with an eye to which ones will bring you in contact with people and activities that feed your sense of aliveness is a way of beginning to assess whether your days are adding up to a joyful life.

Using the joy filter can set in motion a kind of refocusing that tips duty from the center of your life and begins to put happiness and satisfaction in its place. What would happen if, for a day or a week, you cleared your calendar and decided only to refill it with activities that bring you joy?

I'd contend that replacing a to-do list with a joy list would actually allow for more positive results than the familiar ones centered on obligation—and definitely bring more happiness along the way.

Not Selfish. *Necessary.*

It may seem that emphasizing the centrality of joy in later life is petty, selfish, or naive given the suffering that surrounds us in the world and what we face in our own lives. But beauty doesn't disappear because times are hard. The joyful warmth of a loved one's presence doesn't lose its power because it comes when we're ill. Our suffering world can't afford to be without the respite and renewal of the joy we radiate by connecting with a life of meaning.

It's not that we need to slap happy face emojis on every surface. Opening ourselves to joy doesn't mean we won't feel sad, frustrated, furious, or concerned. It means instead that we can find our way back to center and answer despair with sparks of life.

Joy is inside us from the time we're born, ready to be released.

In the years when I worked with patients at the Cancer Research Institute in San Francisco, I used to replenish my emotional reserves almost daily by wandering over to spend time with the joy experts in another part of the hospital: the new fathers and babies in the maternity ward. In those days, babies were separated from their mothers for a time after birth and lined up in cribs behind a large window where family members could stand to see them. Something as simple as a smile or a touch from a nurse could trigger small explosions of delight in those newly minted humans, not to mention those watching, and it was clear that the babies entered this world with a natural capacity for joy.

All these years later, joy can still overtake us. As Joan Chittister writes in *The Gift of Years*: "A blessing of these years is to wake up one morning and find ourselves drunk with the very thought of being alive," something that can turn us into agents of joy who spread it through our world, just like those newborns behind the glass.

Many years ago, when I was in my forties, I had a chance to sit with Norman Cousins, who was then in his wisdom years. As we were discussing the state of the world and ourselves, Norman told me, "Embracing either optimism or pessimism is like voting, like throwing your weight behind a particular outcome when things are still undecided. Why not vote for optimism and put your weight behind a positive outcome since we don't know how things will turn out?"

I know he'd side with joy.

PART TWO

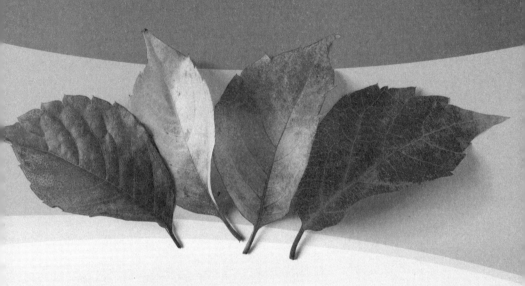

Seeing Your Life

THROUGH

Wisdom's Eyes
and Heart

CHAPTER FOUR

THE FOURTH TASK

Review Your Life to Find Its Patterns and Meaning

"I am astonished, disappointed, pleased with myself.
I am distressed, depressed, rapturous.
I am all these things at once, and cannot add up the sum"

CARL JUNG, *MEMORIES, DREAMS, REFLECTIONS*

W ho are you now? When you stand back and consider the sweep of your life, what do you see? What have you made of the raw material you began with, and what remains to be done?

The Jung quote above appears in the last lines of his autobiographical reflections, and I'm fond of it because it reflects the glorious mess of self that we bring to later life, the complexity that we all carry within us as we move into our sixties and beyond. Our stories by now are filled with contradictory impulses, strengths and failings, confusion and clarity—our deep humanity.

At this stage of life, an impulse builds to somehow make sense of it all and to gaze on the totality of who we are and have been. There may be no simple way to sum up a life, but in over forty years of working with people nearing death, I've seen that as our time grows short, all of us feel an urgency to try. It becomes our paramount task to figure out what it meant that we walked the planet and to seed the future with what we value most. Life review in those late hours is a powerful act that strips away the chaff and lets us see what was most important. Death doesn't let us pretend or look away.

Here at the cusp of the wisdom years, we're contemplating lives that may (or may not) stretch another decade or more if we live beyond eighty-five—the marker of "old-old age." And that gives us an opportunity that doesn't exist on a deathbed. We can pause and take stock while we still have time to address regrets, and show love, forgiveness, and gratitude to those who are most important to us, and act on our deepest wishes.

I've been pondering and reviewing my life a great deal this past decade, starting slowly and without much clarity at about age sixty-five and continuing to the present day—age seventy-five—with far more understanding and depth. I seem to be spending much time lately "going back the way I came" in a search for what has mattered most in my life, the life experiences that have had the greatest impact, the stories that have defined me.

I'm looking for what will serve me well in the time ahead and what I can put aside. To grow past adulthood into wisdom, it helps to examine our narratives, challenging the ones that are no longer true for us, recognizing parts of ourselves that we've hidden or denied. Doing that gives us a more nuanced picture of who we've been, and it can lead us to a liberating sense of self-acceptance. The past is dynamic, alive, and responsive to the new understandings we bring. So is our unwritten future. We have the opportunity, if we take it, to step into a new relationship with ourselves. We can bring to life parts that have lain dormant, and interpret even the most troubling aspects of our lives in ways that give us a sense of peace and hope, freeing our energy for all that is to come.

Some people have likened the transition period between adulthood and later life to a chrysalis stage, in which outgrown parts of our lives and ourselves dissolve, allowing a new sense of identity—what we've been calling the Wise Self—to emerge. Life review can be the core of that process. As we reflect on who we've been and gain a new appreciation of our distinctive path, it becomes easier to feel and follow what's vibrant and alive, letting go of what is not. You can begin that process of introspection by summoning your memories and standing back from your story, watching it unspool as if it were a play unfolding on a stage. I'll show you how best to simply observe both the events and the emotions that surface. Then we'll spend the two chapters that follow "in the chrysalis," doing the deeper emotional work of forgiveness and gratitude and self-acceptance, which have extraordinary power to help us dissolve and transform regrets or lingering emotional pain that have kept us trapped. Done carefully, this self-making work can become a ritual of passage that sends us into our wisdom years able to be more nakedly who we are, amplifying the voice of our soul.

If you're willing to look back at who you've been with soft eyes and an open heart, you'll emerge with strong, bright wings, carried forward with the perspective of your generous, loving Wise Self.

Empathy, Gentleness, and the Senses

Softness and openness are essential for the explorations ahead. Many of us are used to considering our lives through the eyes of a critical adult self, which has a strong tendency to reduce a process like this to a tallying of "sins and wins." But you already know what your inner critic has to say. To connect with more nuanced, transformative insights, I suggest using three tools that will make it easier for you to consider your past in a gentle way and avoid getting stuck in the intellectual/judgment-oriented parts of the brain. Each of these tools will put you in contact with the Wise Self, which is grounded in the body and connected with your spirit.

Begin with Photographs

One simple way to start is by gathering photos of you from your childhood, adolescence, young adulthood, and more recent years. The visible presence of your younger selves makes it difficult to assume that they knew what you do now and could have acted as you would today. It's almost impossible not to soften as you see those earlier faces. Follow your own inclinations as you choose photos, whether you're moved to page through entire albums or just extract a few evocative images that speak to you. If you experienced a trauma or upheaval at some point in your life, it can be useful to find photographs taken both before and after. What you see in the eyes of the faces looking back at you will often reveal emotional truths that are clearer than the stories you've come to tell about that period in narratives smoothed by time. Look, too, for joy and freedom and your own quirky individuality pushing through.

It's hard to keep from softening as you study images of the child you were, the sullen or defiant teenager, the young man or woman of thirty with a baby on one hip, the fifty-year-old with exhausted eyes and a clenched smile. It's even harder to hold on to judgments and blame.

Look, for example, at a photo of the twenty-something who set so many wheels in motion as you were starting out. The twenty-five-year-old who stares back at me was full of energy and confidence. I told people then that I wanted to be Mr. Universe (I was a bodybuilder) and that I was going to get a PhD in mathematics. I'd had success in both areas and believed I could keep climbing inexhaustibly to new heights, yet I knew on some level that neither of those was truly in the cards for me. I can't help but smile at who I thought I was then, so sure of myself and so limited in my ability to see beyond the expected and familiar. I can't help but love the enthusiasm and drive of the very young man I once was, and I wish I could put my arm around his broad shoulders and let him know not to fear the shocks that would soon shake up his sense of what he could be.

We expect to feel some distance from our early selves, but even the forty-year-old in a photo, obsessed with something that may seem unimportant now, and the fifty-year-old who's feeling the burdens of adulthood and the first intimations of mortality, seem removed from who we are today. They're just beginning to discover what comes with reversals and loss, struggles and achievement. And they're still very new to any understanding of the natural rhythms of expansion and contraction, time and chance that will lead them to wisdom.

Look at these images, these earlier selves, with kindness, and let that kind regard for yourself accompany you through all of your explorations of the past.

Use Sensory Cues

As Proust knew well, memory is entwined with the senses. The taste of Morning Thunder tea, the scent of Tibetan rope incense, and the pop of a stereo needle on a vinyl album may transport you viscerally to your college dorm room or first apartment and the dreams and fears that lived in you then.

Your madeleine might be the scent of the lilacs that grew behind your house when you were in grade school or the sight of the fuzzy dice that hung from the mirror of your first car or the songs you played obsessively to get you through a tough stretch of a job or relationship. If you've kept old letters or diaries, seeing a note from a distant time can connect you with a moment, a place, a feeling you'd forgotten. You don't need anything more than your memory and some photos to evoke your past, but if you want to dive deeply into a particular period of your life, gather your own memory-opening "madeleines" and keep them around you—they will draw you closer to who you were.

Fall Back on Grounding Breath

Each time you sit to review your life, take a moment to ground yourself in the safety of the present by closing your eyes and taking several slow, deep breaths as you invite your memories to come. Be guided by gentleness, and know that remembering any difficult times does not require reliving them.

Scholars in the science of aging tell us that we are always writing and rewriting the narrative of our lives, a process that deepens our sense of self until the very end. The point at which we say, "And that's exactly how it was. The past is closed. The End" is the point they label "narrative foreclosure," which shuts down our access to the power of finding ever-new meanings in our own story. The breath—the inspiration—we put into the work of life review isn't meant to fuel nostalgia. It may seem paradoxical, but exploring the past brings our future alive.

So breathe, pull together your photos and perhaps some sensory cues, and then begin.

Time Travel: Gathering Stories

You'll likely find yourself carried by a river of stories as soon as you begin to gather photos, and you might want to structure the process of remembering by moving through the decades, photo by photo, over a course of hours, days, or even weeks. See what comes most vividly to mind as you ask: "Who *was* that person in the picture?" Then let memory take you deeper, outside the confines of the frame. Think about the people and experiences that have shaped you, the choices and beliefs that have defined you, the themes that keep recurring. Make notes if you like—my workshop participants often set aside a notebook for that purpose. This isn't a writing exercise, but many people use it as a basis for writing they'll do later to share their most important stories and discoveries with those they love.

I recently gathered a group of seven friends, whose ages ranged from the late fifties to the late seventies, to review our life stories. We intended to meet just once, but we were all so energized by the process that we wound up meeting six more times. What we realized was that it wasn't enough to remember and repeat the stories we've always told about ourselves. After each of us riffled through our memories, guided by curiosity and intuition, we posed questions to ourselves to prompt new insights. We took care to keep returning to our photos, which always led to stories that led to questions that led to more stories and new realizations about what parts of our pasts wanted our attention now.

It's almost impossible to replicate that kind of freeform process in a book, so the rest of this chapter is divided into sections that pose sets of questions that we found useful, along with the stories they prompted. The nature of memory is meandering, riffing, layered, and I encourage you to wander through your past, exploring the themes that interest you most. Follow what's most compelling to you now, knowing you can return anytime.

The many questions you'll find below are here to spark you, not to overwhelm. I can tell you from experience that any one of them can be the starting point for intimate and revealing conversations should you want to share them with friends or your own life-review gathering.

While you can streamline this process by using the questions to speed you through your life in a long afternoon of exploration, I suggest you give yourself over to remembering for a while. If you've cultivated the practice of spending time daily in your sacred space, consider devoting that period to memory, reflection, and animated chats with your younger selves, seeing where they lead.

Going slowly but steadily through your past gives you a chance to let the feeling of particular times and themes seep into your dreams, musings, and conversations, where questions and revelations are likely to surface. The heart and the listening ear of the Wise Self stitch stories in ways that aren't always linear, so be prepared to leap and circle through time as you revisit old loves, turning points, and well-worn truths about yourself that may be far more malleable than you believed.

You know your story and you live inside it, but as you step back to witness it, guided by curiosity and compassion toward your younger selves, I believe you'll feel the gamut of emotions Jung described: disappointment and dismay, yes, but also astonishment and genuine excitement at the richness of who you've been and are yet to be.

Beginnings: The Map You Were Handed

- Who did your family tell you that you were?
- What "truths" about life and yourself did you absorb from your family?

- How did that shape your choices?

Anyone who's ever spent time with a baby knows that we seem to enter the world with distinct personalities, desires, and temperaments that are evident from our earliest days. But our "original selves" are shaped by our families' perceptions of who we are and ought to be, and we sometimes hold those imprinted images of ourselves as true without ever questioning them. So it can be liberating to conjure up your younger self and compare what you see from the inside with the stories, "legends," and labels that defined you from the outside.

If there was one story from my childhood that defined me to my family—and, for many years, to myself—it was probably the one my mother used to tell (and tell) about my "ambitious nature." One memorable day when I was barely more than a toddler, Mom took me to a nearby park, where I climbed to the top of a small slide and slid down, laughing as she looked on. Eager for more, I ran to my Everest: a giant slide twice as high as the one I had just conquered. I slowly made the steep ascent, rung by metal rung, looking down at the playground moms' concerned faces, determined to get to the top. But as I reached the final rung, my foot slipped and I plunged to the asphalt. Mom rushed to me and wiped blood from my forehead, setting me back on my feet, and once my sobs subsided, she tried to lead me home.

But I wouldn't go.

As Mom loved to tell it, I broke away, ran to the slide, and clambered back up. This time, poised triumphantly at the top, I pushed off and swooped down. Only then would I leave the playground.

"That was you, Charles," Mom liked to say. "You had to go back to that slide and prove you could climb it. You were that way with everything! You had to be first. The best. You had to try the things other kids wouldn't."

That story was more about my mother and her own ambitions for a "special boy" than about me, but hearing it again and again, I made it my own origin story, and let it shape my sense of myself for a long time to come.

Maybe there's a similar story in your family or a label that's stuck since childhood, whether you were the ambitious one, the artist whose first scribbles were masterpieces, the big-hearted one who gave his Christmas toys to a boy who didn't have any, or the colicky baby who's always been "sensitive."

If you find a "defining story" like that, sit with a photo of yourself at that age and ask:

- What part of the story was true?
- What other parts of me did it eclipse?
- Is there another story that captures a part of my younger self that was hidden, private, or secret?

As I think about the little boy who climbed the huge slide and took on the heavy burden of his mother's expectations in the process, I want to let him know that I would embrace him whether he climbed the big ladder or fell and walked away. I want him to know, too, that I treasure a much quieter memory—a series of private, even "secret," memories—that only grow in significance for me as time goes on and continue to reveal more about the boy I was and the man I've become.

On warm nights through my childhood, I loved to sit on our stoop and study the moon, thinking that it grew larger in size even as I watched it, that it leaned toward me as a friend does to whisper a secret. The glowing moon was a soothing presence watching out for me, saying, "Keep your eyes up here and I will guide you." During sad times when I felt lonely and insignificant, the moon offered solace. It promised that there was a pattern in the cosmos, and I was part of it. The moon would be my friend forever.

This isn't something I could tell my parents or brother or friends. I didn't have a way to explain the way looking into the night sky created a mystical and sustaining sense of that connection I felt, and still feel, with something much larger than I am.

"When you grow up, Charlie," I want to tell my younger self, "the moon really will be there for you."

And what does the boy tell me when I listen to him now? "Just because you proved you can do something doesn't mean you have to do it again and again," says the climber. "Sometimes, it feels good just to play ball or eat pancakes. Or sit quiet and rest." (Wisdom indeed for my life now.)

We're used to measuring our lives with dramatic markers, but as you retrace your path, feel for the invisible stories, the moments when you felt most yourself, even—or especially—when no one else could see.

It's particularly interesting, once you've done this, to skip ahead through your life and examine later "defining legends" of your triumphs or character—some chosen or kept alive by you—that may have a way of obscuring as much as they reveal. No one story, no matter how dramatic or glorious, can fully define you.

Dreams: The Lives You Imagined

- What did you dream of being and doing as a child, an adolescent, and in your earlier adult life?
- What's become of your early dreams and fascinations?

- When have you been most fully yourself? What roles or settings freed you?
- What were your soul and imagination calling you to be?
- What does your younger self want you to remember now? Are there promises to that self that you still need to keep?

The rote answers to "What did you want to be when you grew up" sometimes feel pat and practiced. "A pro athlete. A fireman. A mother. A teacher." But often there were tendencies that revealed what felt like the earliest callings or interests that you bent toward like a plant to the sun, but may never have taken seriously. Your photos may remind you of a "phase" worth remembering, a time when something true and important revealed itself or bloomed in you.

"I always say I knew I was a writer from the time I was little," said my workshop student Liz, who indeed has spent her life working with words, mostly at PR firms. "It's easy to tell that story about myself. But I came across an old box of stuff I'd left at my mom's and found a cookbook I made as a kid. I got kind of excited when I sat down and connected all the dots that led from cooking in an EZ-Bake Oven to copying recipes into a notebook and making my own cookbooks, to spending a whole winter looking at a seed catalog and plotting out maps of the garden I wanted to plant. I hadn't thought about that in years. I couldn't get enough of *Little House on the Prairie* and the way the Wilders built and farmed and cooked. When I got to junior high, I fell in love with cooking and sewing in home ec class, as they called it back then.

"My mom hated any kind of homemaking, so she left me alone to play. I made all my own clothes in high school, flowy hippie things that took very little skill. But it made me so happy to be creating myself that way."

Liz told me that when she was in college, she and her boyfriend fantasized about building a handmade house and "living on the land." "But my father grew up poor on a farm and was appalled I wanted to 'go backward,'" she said. "I know it sounds like a hippie fantasy now, and I never really pursued it, but there is something that really appeals to me about making a life by hand, closer to nature. I still love the idea of making our lives into art, making music, making things that seem beautiful and personal, not for sale, but for *life*. I did that when I was younger. I wove things. Wrote poetry. Handmade books. I get excited thinking about it." Her face lit up, then suddenly fell.

When she started working, she said, she didn't know how to bring "my handmade self" into that world. "The fantasy burst, and I just wanted to look like a professional and fit in. I became a kind of workaholic, and fast forward forty years, I don't really do many of those things I loved so much, and haven't for a long time, not even much cooking."

But now she wondered: "What would it feel like to make a delicious dinner or sew up something that's not chic or Instagram perfect but just colorful and one-of-a-kind? Or draw things to put on the walls? Tend some plants?" she said. "Just the thought of it makes me so happy. There's a whole self I don't take out of the box very often."

You may not find a whole vein of abandoned loves as you feel your way back to who you were and wanted to be earlier in your life. But you may come in contact with a feeling you want to carry into later life or get the jolt of energy that comes from being in the presence of a dream that still has power for you, even if so far it has "only" existed in your longings and imagination.

Turning Points: The Choices You Made

- What key events and choices changed the course of your life?
- Which roads not taken are still calling you? Which ones can you leave behind with no regret?

Sometimes looking back, we can pinpoint moments when our hearts wanted to say yes, or no, to an opportunity or direction, but our heads said the opposite. In our life-review group, we found that sometimes old longings and directions still called to us and that our stories of turning away from them brought up raw feelings of regret. Just as often, though, we found that a gust that seemed to blow us off course had actually led to a relationship, choice, or move that in retrospect felt like destiny. Our younger selves tended to view turning points as either/or, black/white points of no return, and we reminded each other as we listened that we may yet write new endings.

Beth, the accountant, looked back at her younger selves with sadness. She had always wondered what would have happened if she'd followed her love of animals and built her life around that love. As she reviewed her life, she saw once again how animals had been a touchstone of the childhood stories that were most vivid to her. "From the time I was tiny, I would follow cats down the street and want to bring them home. I begged for a puppy, and when someone gave us a little Easter duckling, I fed it in the back yard till my father took it away. I told everyone I was going to be a vet when I grew up."

She rescued stray cats, nursed injured birds back to health, and rushed to the coast in high school to try to save oil-covered animals after an oil spill. She was *sure* she was meant to be a vet. But when it came time for her to graduate from high school, her father told her he'd only pay for college if she entered a business program. "You can love animals all you want," he said, "but they're not going to pay your bills.

People will always need an accountant. You need to be able to take care of yourself first." Her eyes teared up as she told me, "I don't know why I didn't put up more of a fight. It's not exactly that I blame myself for not insisting, but I feel as though I betrayed myself in that moment and gave up the life I was supposed to have. It was a huge turning point."

One way of facing old losses like this, I told her, is to spend time with the still-active emotions, working to channel the potent energy of sadness or regret into outlets that reflect the passion that's never subsided. A turning point that was once a "turning away," like Beth's, can be revisited in later life and spark a "turning toward" what's been neglected.

Tara, a woman in our life-review group who's in her late sixties, focused on a turning point that was less a single moment than a question that had hung over her life for many years: Should she have become a mother? Tara knew without a doubt in her twenties that she wanted to be her own woman, able to fly high, roam the world, and experience the best life had to offer. "I wanted to live high on the hog," she said with a smile. She came of age reading *The Feminine Mystique* and decided to "be a feminist my own way," by getting an MBA and becoming a retail consultant in the fashion industry. "That was my independent streak," she said. "I wanted to make a statement simply by succeeding. And I didn't want to be tied to the needs of a husband and kids or follow somebody else's agenda. It was important to me to do exactly what I wanted to, which was a pretty radical idea."

She acknowledged that while she would've denied it at the time, her mother had had more than a little influence over her decision. "Mom was sharp and ambitious, but she was bullied by the expectations of her time. She didn't go to college—she got a job as an executive secretary, which she loved. And then she wound up marrying one of her bosses," Tara told us. "Dad wanted her to stay home with us, and she did, but she always resented being a housewife and mom. When I was growing up, she always told me, 'Your independence is everything! I wish I'd stayed single and never had kids,' which I admit is a pretty harsh thing to say to one of your own children."

Tara thrived as a consultant, sans husband or kids. "There's just one thing that has haunted me," she said. "When I hit my mid-thirties and could hear my biological clock ticking, I wondered if I was just living out my mother's dreams and not my own. Even though I have loved my life, and I thought I'd made peace with staying single and childless, I guess I'm still struggling with that decision."

Most of the women in our group came of age at a moment when entering the workforce felt like a revolutionary act, and motherhood seemed like a choice that would bind them to a traditional role they didn't want. Now we talked about the gifts and sacrifices wrapped up in that choice and the ways they had expressed mothering in their lives, and still could. Tara knew she'd want to spend more time sitting with her Wise Self, considering what she'd chosen at that crossroads. (We'll do further work with regret in the chapters ahead.)

Love, Joy, and Satisfaction
- What astonishes you as you look back?
- What work or activity has given you the greatest sense of pride and satisfaction?
- Who and what have you loved the most?
- Whose love has meant the most to you?
- What's brought you the greatest joy?
- What are you most grateful for in your life?

I've listened to many people review their pasts as their days grew short, wondering about the meaning of their lives. What I noticed is that for all the energy we put into concerns about success or status or wealth or comfort as we race through life, the truth I heard repeatedly is summed up in this quote from President Barack Obama: "In the fleeting time we have on this earth, what matters is not wealth, or status, or power, or fame, but rather, how well we have loved, and what small part we have played in making the lives of other people better."

The set of questions above will help to remind you of what is of the most value in your life, and how much energy you've given to what matters most to you. The stories that come now can reflect back to you the parts of your life that have been most fulfilling, and it can be refreshing simply to linger here, savoring the best of your life so far and orienting yourself toward "more of this"—whether what you're seeing is kindness, courage, beauty, love, or the honoring of a gift that is entirely private and unique to you, the particular human qualities you bring to the rest of humanity.

"The thing that most astonishes me, and gives me great satisfaction and joy, has to do with a decision I made when I was forty-two to 'follow my bliss,'" Carla, a life coach in her late sixties, told our life-review group. "My parents grew up in the Depression, and the most important thing to them was security. They drilled into me the idea that education was my ticket to the kind of life I deserved. They were so proud when I graduated from college and then law school. It was a miracle to them, and such a relief. I went into corporate litigation, the jungle. We were formidable, and I was the queen of billable hours, working my way up to partner.

"So you're looking at me like, what?" she said with a laugh. "People I meet these days don't even know about that part of my life. Because it was a big detour from who I really am. From the time I was a child, I wanted to help people who were suffering, and I could've done that in law. But when I took on those huge student loans, I felt I had to be realistic. I couldn't spend all that money and come out the other end a public defender or crusader. So I didn't. I went straight for white-shoe corporate law. And I won't lie. I was extremely proud of my success and being able to make enough to send my folks on vacations and make their lives more comfortable."

But when she hit her early forties, Carla realized she was mostly handling cases in which "I couldn't pretend I was working for the good guys," and she felt increasingly uneasy and depressed. "I knew I'd chosen wrong. My job offered money and power and status. But the work also diminished me, and left me with the feeling that I'd stopped listening to my conscience, my heart. I didn't like who I was becoming. I wanted to help people, not companies, and do it in a direct way. I guess that was my midlife crisis."

When she heard about a new profession called life coaching, she knew immediately that that's what she wanted to do. It wasn't therapy; it was focused on helping people "thrive in lives that fit"— and that's exactly what she knew she needed to do, both for herself and her future clients. "Without being totally conscious of it, I realized that I was not willing to go to my deathbed knowing that I'd denied what was right for me," she said. So despite her fear of making such a drastic change, and the alarm of her family and colleagues, she quit her job to get a life-coaching certificate. "I never felt so liberated in my life," she said. "It was pretty rough going at times—when I said I was a coach, people thought I meant sports—but I felt like I had given birth to my real self, and I could serve other people by helping them to do the same."

Her joy was infectious, and we leaned forward to take it in. Now, more than twenty years later: "I'm still so grateful and amazed that I found the courage to take a chance on myself, and I feel as though I have been living my dream," she said. She paused. "The interesting thing as I say this is that I realize I've been hearing a little voice inside recently that makes me wonder if there might be a different next chapter for me. Maybe not far from what I'm doing, but not the same, either. A lot of my joy came from taking a chance on that little voice . . ."

Carla, coach that she was, reminded us that even the path that satisfied us the most through our adult lives might, and probably will, give way to the callings of an older, wiser body and soul in later life. Attuning ourselves to what's brought joy can sensitize us to the *feeling* of joys we haven't yet recognized.

Carl, a quiet man in his early seventies, described the quieter satisfactions of his own deep loves.

"What really comes to the front of my mind when I think about what I love in my life is people—I guess that's natural to say. People and books. I toiled away at my job in tech support, which put food on the table for most of my adult life, but my refuge and comfort has always been reading. My sister was born premature when I was five, and she's struggled with lingering health and emotional issues. She's fragile even now. My job as a kid was to take care of myself so my mom could focus on her. And that's where books came in. I may have been alone a lot, but I wasn't lonely—I was a good reader, having adventures on Treasure Island. Books and my imagination were my best friends.

"When I got older, I would stop off at our local bookstore after school. Other kids hung out at an ice cream place down the block, but I couldn't walk past the book display without going in. I hardly ever bought anything, but the owner was so kind. He let me sit there reading in a back aisle almost every afternoon, never rushing me out, always saying hello and commenting on what he saw me pick up. I don't know why he was so kind. In a way, he took me in. I've always been grateful for the way he made me part of his tribe of book lovers, his family."

Carl's other great love is his wife Ana, a fellow bibliophile he met on a blind date. "I thought I'd always be alone—I didn't meet Ana until I was an old bachelor of fifty-five—but her laughter and curiosity and friends pulled me into the world," he said. "I still can't get over the way she's always loved me for who I am, even when I act like a guy who's spent way too much time by himself. She made me believe in love. I don't know how I've been so lucky in my life. There have been a lot of things that haven't worked out the way I wanted. Tough stuff with my family, my job. But I have a lot of joy. When I get down on myself, I try to remember just what a lucky man I am. I always go home to Ana and our books."

What joys stand out for you? Spend time savoring the memories, absorbing their energy.

Difficulty, Disappointment, Obstacles

- Is there anything that leaves you with a lingering sense of anger, resentment, guilt, or shame?
- What do you regret most in your life?
- Where have fears and obstacles arisen, and how have you faced them?
- What still weighs on you from your past? Are there secrets that burden you?
- Is there anyone, including yourself, you need to forgive?

I know that taking stock of the tough parts of life can bring out the well-honed critical voice of the adult self. As you consider the threads of disappointment, obstacles, and difficulties in your stories, it's helpful to actively tame the tendency to beat up on yourself or fire up old emotions. You can use your photos to good effect by letting them help you reconnect with the younger selves. Remember that those versions of yourself couldn't, and didn't, have the level of emotional maturity and wisdom that it's taken you a lifetime to earn.

All too often we judge missteps, shortcomings, and failures— even the smallest ones—as evidence of irredeemable flaws. But please don't view any regret or remorse you feel now as invitations for self-flagellation. See them for what they are: clues to what's been left unsaid, undone, unactualized, unappreciated, unforgiven—a starting point for the soul work of later life.

As you reflect on the questions above, note what comes. Keep in mind that we'll continue to work with the stories that come up here.

In our life-review group, the discussion of regrets hovered around a few big themes: Relationships, often with our parents, children, or exes, that had left us with unresolved pain, guilt, or resentment. Memories of hurts we'd inflicted, apologies we'd never made. Times we'd stayed too long with the wrong person or a job that was wrong for us. Disappointment that we'd spent our lives playing it safe and never taken a chance on our big dreams. Fears that it was too late to change.

For Carl, many of those issues came together as he described his regrets about a road not taken. "So it's not going to surprise you that I actually had, I mean *have*, a dream that involves books," he told us. "I got all the way to my forties telling myself that I'd done pretty well in my job and was making a good living. But it started to bother me that my best friends, Clark and Fred, who I knew from temple, were always talking about how much they loved their jobs and even seemed *excited* about going to work—and I didn't. One day I mentioned that to Fred and he asked me, 'What is it that *you* would love to do?' Without thinking, I told him that I wanted to open a bookstore/coffee house where people could hang out and read; a community that revolved around books. I don't think I'd admitted to myself that I wanted to do that, but there it was.

"That's supposed to be the end of the story, the way it was for Carla—she sees what she needs to do, and voilà! Next thing you know, she's a life coach instead of a lawyer. But that's not how it was for me." Carl paused and his eyes watered. "I didn't have the guts to quit my career. I wasn't rich, but I had health insurance and paid vacations and I could save for retirement, which I'm pretty damn glad about now. I was making my parents proud—more than anything they wanted me to 'have a secure future' and they loved it that I was at IBM. But I'm not proud of that, not really. And I know it's wrong, but I kind of resent them for training me so well to do what *they* wanted me to do instead of encouraging me to be myself. The thing I really regret is that I was always too timid to act in support of my dream.

"I went into therapy for a time and even went to my rabbi for advice about this when I was in my fifties. And do you know what everyone told me? 'Try it! Why not give your dream a chance?' Ana has patiently listened for the past fifteen years, and she's always said, 'It'll happen when you're ready.' I was never ready enough to try. I feel as though I've disappointed myself, and her, too.

"So that's the dark side of my happy life," he said after a long pause. "I'd really like to escape into a book right now instead of thinking about it, but I think what I'm feeling is good. If I'm going to do this, it's kind of now or never. Maybe it won't be a bookstore, exactly, but something in that world. I'm just so afraid that I won't have the guts to do it before I die. I don't fully trust myself to do it, but this regret is eating me up."

Heads nodded, and we spoke about how we all deserve the chance to live our own lives and how something within us protests when we're not doing so, when we hide from ourselves and choose safety, comfort, and security rather than authenticity.

Later life isn't typically described as a time of risk-taking, but we have the time, depth, and experience, now, to take the biggest risk of our lives, to move beyond regret and, perhaps for the first time in many years, to allow ourselves to be guided toward our deepest dreams, aided by the clarity that comes from a life review.

As you reflect on who you've been and what you've done to date in your life, know that you are giving yourself the opportunity to celebrate the collective growth of all the younger selves that look out from the photos in front of you. Our lives are complex, mystifying, astonishing. I know that joy and disappointment exist side by side with your wildest hopes and the burgeoning vision of who you are now, feeling the callings of your wisdom years. Please sit with all that, letting insights bloom.

Time spent in the chrysalis of emotional work will help you address any regret, remorse, or pain that's been surfacing and reconnect you with a sense of gratitude to carry you forward. Take that time.

CHAPTER FIVE

THE FIFTH TASK

Do the Heart-Opening
Work of Forgiveness

I t's gratifying to do the hard work of reviewing the past, regarding yourself from a distance to appreciate who you've been, what you've made of the raw materials of your life, what you've learned and overcome.

And yet, sometimes what lingers after a life review is the painful memory of wrongs and shortcomings, guilt and stings, betrayals and disappointments, ways you and others inflicted harm or didn't measure up. You can be swamped by difficult emotions that overwhelm the joy that comes with connecting to the essence of who you are.

But you don't have to stay there. In our competitive, ego-driven adult years, we're often in the grip of a strong need to be right and keep score in relationships, which feeds a sense of being aggrieved, let down, or owed. In later life, though, we're increasingly conscious of the cost of staying locked in old battles, no matter how right we may be. The price of harsh self-judgment becomes clear as well. "Are you sure you want to wall off your heart instead of making room for compassion?" the Wise Self asks. To which Death, the pithiest of advisers adds, "Do you really want to spend the time you have left replaying and judging your life instead of living it?"

Both of these advisers counsel forgiveness, though they're not talking about wiping the slate clean and pretending that a painful or harmful episode never happened. True forgiveness, the kind that transforms us and brings us peace, has several components:

- the release of anger, guilt, resentment, and disappointment connected to being wronged,
- the giving-up of the desire to punish another person or oneself,
- and the acknowledgment of the complex mix of positive and negative that all of us share because we're human.

This can be some of the most challenging work of the chrysalis time, bringing us face-to-face with issues, people, and aspects of ourselves that we may have pushed to the periphery so we could "get on with our lives." That's the illusion—that we can resolve the pain of old emotional injuries by burying them under activity, distraction, or silence. But my end-of-life work has shown me how steadily the longing for compassion and honorable closure builds around old wounds when they're left untended. Those who have delayed asking for and offering forgiveness until the very end urgently seek the peace it brings and are liberated by releasing the hurts of the past. So are we all as we learn to forgive.

Forgiveness is a central task of later life, and it comes more naturally to us now because age and experience are beginning to create a kind of softening of the heart, a melting into a larger, more gracious self. By the time we get to sixty or seventy we know that nobody's perfect, or can be—least of all ourselves. All of us have hurt and betrayed others. All of us have hurt and betrayed ourselves. And all of us have felt the sting of being hurt and betrayed. There is much to forgive and much that connects us to the rest of humanity as we acknowledge our common frailty and failings, the pain all of us have shared. It's easier to see the many shades of gray in our lives now, especially after doing a life review. The black-and-white assessments that may have prevailed earlier seem less complete, less absolute, as we step into our wisdom years.

A fear we may carry is that if we let the old hurts lose their intensity, it will mean that we have forgotten them, betraying our earlier selves. But to forgive does not mean to forget or condone or minimize what happened. It doesn't require reconciliation—that's not the goal. Forgiveness is a decision to let go of past grievances because holding onto them causes suffering that cuts us off from the present, where we can heal and learn and love.

We can forgive by ourselves, for our own peace of mind, without requiring anything of others. We can choose to do it because it reduces our reactiveness and changes the way we regard a situation that may not objectively change at all. We can choose to forgive to give ourselves a new start and regain the capacity to trust. We can choose it because, as our Wise Self knows, all that's in our power to change is ourselves. We can forgive quietly, without saying a word to the party we have forgiven. And with forgiveness, we can powerfully rewrite the narrative of our lives and expand our sense of peace.

Whom Do You Need to Forgive?

If you're like the people in my workshops and life-review group, you probably know exactly where to target forgiveness work. See what leapt to mind when you asked yourself the final series of questions in the last chapter, especially these:

- Is there anything that leaves you with a lingering sense of anger, resentment, guilt, or shame? (Also ask: Is there a person who still gets you angry or irritated or upset?)
- What do you regret most in your life?
- Is there anyone, including yourself, you need to forgive?

It often happens that the need to forgive and the need to be forgiven—whether by another person or ourselves—are closely bound, and the relief that comes from one spills into a desire for the other. Whatever your starting point, it's almost certain that you'll wind up working toward both. Let your soul and psyche tell you where to focus right now, as Death asks you this highly clarifying question: "If you knew you had just a few months to live, who would you forgive or ask forgiveness of? And what would you forgive your younger self for?"

Take a moment to breathe and reflect on what comes up.

The stories below, drawn from my life and from participants in my workshops and life-review group, will walk you through some essential components of forgiveness in some of the layered situations we face in later life. Forgiveness doesn't happen instantly, though there are tools and attitudes that can help make it easier. It's an ongoing process that can, with practice, become a way of being that nourishes and begins to define you in your wisdom years. In my groups and workshops, we have all found that the more energy we put into releasing our old perceptions of and reactions to the past, the more energy we free. If your "forgiveness list" is long, know that the potential for relief is only that much greater.

Chain Reactions: Old Stories, Old Responses

Tara, the fashion industry consultant in our life-review group, came to one of our meetings after spending a weekend with her mother. "It really brought up, once again, how much I need to resolve things with her," Tara said. "I was helping her do some things around the house, and she took me down to the basement to show me something she wanted to give me, some fabric she got in Europe years ago. It was gorgeous, and I thanked her not just for the gift but for being part of the reason I got into fashion. It seemed like a rare happy moment between us. But of course, it didn't last long.

"Looking through the chest, I pulled out something I'd never seen before, a souvenir pillow from Niagara Falls—from her honeymoon! I had never even known they went to Niagara Falls. I begged her for the story, but that just made her angry. 'I should have thrown that thing away,' she told me. But she finally did say more. She said she cried on her honeymoon and wanted to go home, but she didn't think her family would take her back. Then she looked at me and said, 'I never should have married your father. It's the worst decision I ever made. I never should have done it. And I never should have had kids. It ruined my life.'

"It's not like it was a surprise," Tara said. "I've heard that my whole life. You have to understand that she'll often say, 'You're the best thing that ever happened to me,' and in almost the same breath she'll say, 'I wish I'd never had kids.' That's the way she's always been. 'I love you, let me give you something nice, but by the way, you ruined my life.' I feel like I've got pretty thick skin by now, but sometimes it really hurts. I know she's old, and I don't think she always realizes the effect of her words, but it just makes me crazy. And angry."

Tara realized she'd been talking faster and faster, and she paused to take a deep breath.

"I left home as soon as I could and got far away from her. I've been realizing that I've lived a lot of my life in reaction to her. She had kids and resented it, and I decided not to have kids of my own, but since my life review I've been wondering once again if I did the right thing." She sighed. "Mom can still push that button and raise my blood pressure in nothing flat. I'm ashamed to say that when she started talking about regretting getting married and having a family, I snapped at her and said, 'Stop talking like that!' And then I stormed out like a teenager. People wonder why I don't call and visit her all the time now that she's eighty-five. Well, that's why. The thing is, I don't want to be that teenager anymore. I know Mom needs me and I'm letting her down. I'm so tired of being blamed when she feels unhappy. But I'm tired also of getting sideswiped by this crazy rage and resentment that I didn't get a different mother."

A First Step: Externalizing the Emotions

The goal of forgiveness is to bring ourselves peace. And peace is hard to come by when our accounts of old hurts and grievances are cycling through us in closed loops that feed themselves in the retelling, throwing new instances of the hurt like logs on a fire and keeping difficult emotions burning hot. For Tara, words she heard as "You ruined my life" were such a painful and familiar refrain that they could overpower the generous moments of any call or visit.

It's helpful—essential even, in cases like Tara's—to take the painful stories out of your head and bring them into a space where you can begin to witness the troubling situation, including your feelings, from the vantage point of an outside observer. I often recommend that people do this by talking with a trusted friend or counselor who can listen from the heart, give deep attention to your words and body language, and receive them with compassion.

Let this person know that you don't want advice. What's more helpful and desirable is the perspective of a neutral party who can listen to the whole story as you detail your experiences and emotions.

It's obviously not a good idea to choose a person who's been hearing your grievances for years and played the role of faithful partisan; you're looking for a kind, unbiased listener who is willing to point out what he or she notices about what's going on, including the part you've played in the situation. This person's questions and observations can help you see this familiar emotional terrain in a new way.

It's important to set aside time to do this. We can't shortcut the deep, honest, emotional work that true forgiveness requires. It's necessary first to wade courageously into what still roils us and acknowledge the feelings that still flare from old wounds—including the grief that comes with longing for things to have been different, and the anger and indignation of believing we deserved better or were robbed of innocence, protection, or hope. It's crucial to *examine* those thoughts and emotions, not suppress them, and to stay with the process of looking, questioning, and noticing.

Talking things out with another person—not stepping into a cycle of venting and escalation but bringing hurtful memories into the light and looking with curiosity at what happened to those familiar characters in your story—can give you new clarity both about the events and how you have interpreted and responded to them.

Tara told me later that she'd found a helpful listener in a friend from her longtime book group. "I've always admired the way Julia seems to take in everything and come back with comments that show

how carefully she's been paying attention. I really trusted that she'd be able to hear what I was saying and help me get some perspective.

"As I told her my story, she noticed the way Mom likes to have an antagonist, whether it's my father or me or my brothers, someone to blame for whatever makes her unhappy. And she noticed how crazy that makes me. She also pointed out to me how often I start to say positive things—like how touched I was when Mom wanted to give me that beautiful fabric or how much I appreciate that she held things together in our family when my dad couldn't—but then I pull back into old hurts and start fighting with her again.

"Julia said something, almost in passing, like 'It seems like you two really have a hard time saying "I love you" without bringing in your mom's regrets.' And she was so right. This has been going on for sixty-six years! It surprised me that she was so moved when I told her about Mom and the honeymoon pillow. 'She must've been so sad and scared,' Julia said, 'but she kept the pillow all these years. She didn't throw it away.' I realized how hard-hearted I get around Mom. A wall goes up so I won't get hurt, but that hurts both of us. I can't see my mom as a person, and she can't really see me," Tara said. "Julia pointed out how Mom and I are both trying to do good things for each other. She said she wondered what would happen if I could somehow stay focused on that instead of getting sucked into Mom's blaming and regrets. I've been thinking about that, wondering what it would take."

A Second Step: Pivoting Away from the Old Reactions by Using AND

Forgiveness starts with *wanting* to forgive, wanting the peace that forgiveness can bring. As Tara talked with her friend, she had a chance to see not only the long-term patterns at play but also her own desire to be free of her automatic reactions, the seemingly inevitable slide into anger and sadness that came when she was with her mother. Externalizing your emotions and getting feedback from a compassionate listener isn't a magic cure for old angers and resentments. The hurt is still there, and it often has the freshness and power that come from being recently fed. But stepping into an observer's role can make it possible to ask, "What if?" What if you chose another way to respond?

One thing I'd suggest is that it's possible to choose new responses that cultivate forgiveness, even as you acknowledge the old feelings that still exist.

It's not necessary to wait until the feelings are gone. Instead, we can do two seemingly opposite things simultaneously: feel and tend the hurt of the old feelings AND shift our attention and energy toward thoughts and actions that can bring us peace. Taking the "AND" view of reality breaks through the impasse that comes from believing that the other person, or the pain in our heart, must change before we can alter our responses in the present moment. We can live in the complexity, and the possibilities, of who we are now.

Here are some examples of AND formulations that helped Tara and other members of my groups hold this "tension of opposites" and move toward forgiveness.

- I'm disappointed and hurt AND I'm willing to set aside the need to hurt the other person in return. I'm willing to do this for my own well-being.
- I know I'm in the right AND I'm willing to consider that even in wronging me or letting me down, the other person did the best they could with the inner and outer resources they had at the time.

- I'm hurt by the other person's words AND I realize that I may have something to do with provoking their anger when I speak without thinking.
- I'm angry AND I'm willing to honestly consider my part in the situation as it exists today.
- I'm angry/hurt/resentful about the past AND I'm willing to see that the other person and I are not the same as we were long ago. Both of us have changed. I'm willing to look at this situation through the eyes of the person I am today.
- I'm deeply hurt AND I'm willing to acknowledge that I was not uniquely singled out for this injustice; what happened to me happens to countless others. I'm not being persecuted. What I'm facing/have faced is part of being an imperfect human in an imperfect world.
- I'm upset because my head wants a different outcome than the one I got AND I'm willing to listen to my heart, which wants to respond to the situation with kindness and love.
- I carry the hurts and scars of my relationship with someone AND I'm willing to act with kindness and love anyway.

Each of the AND statements helps unfreeze the situation by adding a larger perspective or way of responding to the status quo. These can sit as possibilities within us, allowing us to pause, breathe, and access the emotional intelligence we have in later life, focusing on who we are and what we want now.

The Kids on the Seesaw

Turning your attention to the AND statements helps bring the mind and emotions into balance. You could liken it to riding a seesaw. Before we try to forgive, there is only a long list of hurts, and each time an old story is repeated or a new grievance is added, it's as though another kid piles onto the resentment end of the seesaw. Nothing can move. The load just gets heavier and heavier, more earthbound. Stuck. But pivoting away from the hurt with an AND gives emotional weight and reality to a counterbalancing possibility. Yes, there's been pain and ugliness, but it doesn't preclude the presence of beauty. A history of hurt doesn't have to crush our present-day impulses toward kindness or love. It can, instead, give greater meaning to the choice to move toward love. Our lives are both/and, not either/or. And we can put the weight of our attention and behavior on what we have the power to change—our responses in the present.

- "I realized that what's true for me is that I'm a loving person, and anger is a big issue for me when I'm around my mom," Tara told me. "I saw that we tend to egg each other on. So I'm making a conscious effort not to feed the beast. I don't really want to have the same old arguments about who's right about the past and who's to blame.

- "I had a couple of sessions with my old therapist, who helped me come up with a few neutral things to say that don't throw gasoline on the fire. If Mom is critical or blaming, I don't argue. I say, 'I'm sorry you feel that way.' Period. Or I say, 'I'm glad you had me, Mom. Let's talk about the good times.' Or, 'Mom, we all did the best we could with what we knew at the time.' I even say, 'I love you.' If she says something that stings, I try to take a deep breath and say, "Ouch! That hurt," and stop there. Those few lines are my entire script when she gets into regrets and blaming. I don't add anything. I just let it sit. It's been kind of funny. I still have some sadness and frustration, and I wish we'd had a happier family life. But

I'm getting better at being with her as she is, and we don't get sucked into the swamp as much. She's starting to say back to me, 'Let's talk about the good times,' and we do. I didn't think it could happen."

In pivoting away from old reactions to old hurts, even when it feels stilted to consciously switch the script, we can find ourselves softening and our feelings shifting. Tara noticed that she'd been starving her relationship with her mother of love while waiting to be loved, and the decision to forgive—to consciously pause her habitual armored and angry responses and allow other possibilities in—brought longed-for warmth into her dealings with her mom and a dramatic lessening of resentments.

A key for me in my life was realizing that my parents did the best they could, given how they were raised and who they became as a result. They did very well in some ways and not so well in others— which is precisely the same as the rest of us. Realizations like this can bring empathy and perspective as well as, for some of us, an increased capacity for forgiveness, love, and compassion for those who we previously felt had hurt us.

We often speak of forgiveness as "letting go" of painful feelings. Jack Kornfield, the noted mindfulness teacher, helpfully explains: "To let go does not mean to get rid of. To let go means to let be. When we let be with compassion, things come and go on their own." We can compassionately notice the pain and allow ourselves, and our relationship with the other person, to be larger than just that.

The Way It Might Have Been versus the Way It Is

We don't want old wounds to weigh us down during our final years, when our strongest desire is to give and fulfill and be our largest, most genuine selves. As we learn to forgive, we prove that we're capable of growing and learning and healing and loving. And when we realize we can finally forgive others for not meeting our hopes and expectations, we realize that we can also forgive ourselves—often for things that happened years ago—and ask for forgiveness from those we've hurt.

Lena, a woman in one of my groups a while back, spoke movingly about the way her life as a parent had been full of unmet expectations of herself and her son Tim. She'd had a polite but strained relationship with him for many years and longed to be closer, even as she pushed down her hopes that anything could change. Tim had always been her "special child," the one she knew was destined for greatness from the time he was tiny. "He was extremely bright, a genius we thought, with a great personality," she said. "He was a star at everything he did from sports to school to friendships, and we were sure he'd be a tremendous success." She had dreams that he'd become a doctor or lawyer, and her husband Al, a professor at a large university, was confident that Tim would find his way into academia.

But, as so often happens in families, the son didn't follow his parents' script. "As I look back on it now, it seems as if the more we pushed, the more Tim went the other way," Lena told us. "In high school, he completely rebelled. He quit all his teams and spent all his time making silly little movies. He took theater and art and media studies, but he wouldn't touch the college prep classes he needed, even though they would've been easy for him. Al managed to get him into the college where he works, but Tim said he wanted to travel with his girlfriend. He went one semester and then dropped out."

After that, Tim kept his distance. "He did do some traveling, then found a job and moved in with a lot of other kids. He managed to get by, with our help," Lena said. "He got a job as a temporary secretary where he said he could write between answering phones. He's always blamed us for pushing him too hard and not accepting him for who he is. He doesn't want to live a life like ours, or be anything like us, even if that means sacrificing his talents." Lena paused. "I have spent most of my adulthood feeling like I failed as a parent and wondering how things went so wrong."

Lena said she'd done her best to make peace with the situation. "I get it that Tim had to go his own way and that I can't change that. I don't butt in. I call him on his birthday and send money when I think he needs it. But I don't really have my son in my life." Her voice trailed off. "How did this happen? What did we miss when he was young? I keep asking myself what we could've done differently. I'm afraid for him. What will he do when we're gone? Will he blow his inheritance on dumb things? Will he be a temp or something his whole life? What kind of life is that?"

As we talked about forgiveness in the group, Lena realized that "making peace" by keeping her distance and blaming herself weren't the same as forgiveness. She wasn't sure whom she needed to forgive. Tim? Herself? All she knew was that pushing the problem away only intensified the pain and estrangement, and she didn't want that anymore. She wanted to find a way to rebuild her relationship with her son.

For Lena, as for Tara, finding a compassionate listener was key to moving toward that. She told me later that she'd had a breakthrough when she talked with a trusted older friend to help her sort out her feelings. Her friend listened to her guilt and her worries about Tim's future and said, "You know, Tim's an adult. Have you ever asked him what he plans to do?"

"I began to see how I'd been so focused on my own guilt and disappointment that I never really thought about Tim as an adult or his own person," Lena said. She decided to call him, for the first time in many months, and broach what had been on her mind for so long. Lena and her friend worked out the wording of her questions so they would sound like questions, not accusations, and then she made the call.

Tim was surprised to hear from her. "Stunned is more like it," Lena said. He was guarded at first, but as they talked, he seemed genuinely pleased that she called. "I didn't realize how much I didn't know," she said. "He's at a nonprofit where he works with kids—some kind of program doing theater and helping them make movies—this was the first I heard of it. And he's got a girlfriend he met there. They're doing okay. More than okay. He sounds happy! My old anxiety got the better of me and I kept asking if he had enough money. He got pretty upset. But when I relaxed, he actually joked around, and I remembered how truly funny and creative he is. I've really missed him."

Where We Were Unskilled, We Can Learn

Lena's friend suggested that it might help her to talk to a therapist about the anxiety she had about Tim's ability to fend for himself. She's been taking the time to do just that. As she asks the questions that come more easily to us in later life, she is finding her way toward a new understanding of what happened in her family. Questions such as:

- What were those experiences really about?
- What can I do now to ease my burden and that of the other person?

- How would my life improve if we reconciled, even if it was just in my own mind?

She's been asking, "What's my part in this?" As she explores that question, she's finding it particularly helpful to have support while coming to terms with her role in the rift with Tim—without beating herself up.

Few of us were malicious in our painful dealings with our children, partners, and friends. But we did sometimes hold unrealistic expectations of them, and often of ourselves, and we frequently lacked the skills we needed to listen, empathize, and weather disagreements in constructive ways. Some of us, reared in families where "the parents are always right," never learned the art of give-and-take between parents and kids; while we were expected to say "I'm sorry" when we upset our elders, we may never have heard our parents say those words to us. We may have taken that experience into our own parenting and close interactions. But now we have the opportunity to choose different strategies and act with deeper emotional intelligence. We've got the resources and will to admit our shortcomings, to make apologies, to offer and ask for forgiveness. And if we still lack the skills to do that, we can learn—and grow into a new relationship with the past.

"The tough thing to admit is that we really *were* trying to get him to live the life we wanted, so we'd be 'successful parents,' and for as much as I thought I was always thinking about him, I worried a lot about what people thought of us," Lena admitted. "I lost track of *Tim*—what he really wanted, who he was. I stopped asking. The thing is, he's pretty darn successful on his own terms. He's doing what he wants, he's in love, he's helping people. And I couldn't see any of that because I told myself for so long that if he wasn't a doctor or lawyer, he couldn't possibly be okay."

Once she could see her own actions more clearly, Lena realized she wanted to apologize to Tim for her part in letting such distance come between them and for being so unskilled at managing her expectations of him and of herself. "I had no idea what to do when he turned out to have a mind of his own," she said. "I pushed him in the direction I wanted him to go, and when he said that wasn't what he wanted, I didn't really try to understand. I took it as defiance and rejection, and I retreated and worried. Sometimes I think I tried to buy love with checks.

"I want him to know I'm sorry for all the hurt that I caused, and for saying I was disappointed in him. Tim didn't fail as a son. I'm so proud that he's always insisted on being his own man and succeeding on his own terms, not mine or anyone else's. He's a good person. I've never stopped loving him, though I didn't show that well. I hope he can forgive me and that we can get to know each other again and be closer."

After practicing with her therapist, Lena offered Tim her apology at lunch, using words much like the ones she shared with me. It can be very helpful to have the support of a professional if you long to ask someone for forgiveness and feel stuck or stymied, but many of us do this on our own with great success and relief. These guidelines can be a starting point.

- Take responsibility for your actions. That's the first step when asking for forgiveness, and it starts with clear-eyed awareness and acknowledgment of how you hurt someone (or yourself).

- Then comes the actual apology—"I'm really sorry"—to the person you feel you have wronged followed by an explanation (not belabored) of your actions or omissions (without excuses).
- Show that you feel for the other person by expressing empathy and try to make things right if you can. Ask: What can I do to make things up to you?
- Finally, at least twice, ask simply for the other person's forgiveness.

If you caused injury to your child when he or she was young, it can be healing to tell your adult child: "It wasn't your fault." Those four words can go far in alleviating the self-blame that your child may have carried for a lifetime for something out of his or her control—your divorce, changes in the family's fortunes, even a family member's illness or death. Where there was extreme turmoil in the family—instances of abuse or neglect, or the fallout of a parent's addiction or absence—the most healing action you can take, if you haven't already, is to seek counseling and the support of an appropriate twelve-step program.

It's worth asking for forgiveness even if you don't get it. In fact, asking for forgiveness is the first step toward forgiving yourself—even if the other person isn't ready to respond the way you hoped. It teaches us that we don't always get what we want, even though we might still get what we need. Lena said that what she wants more than being right, more than a superficial, distant peace with her son, is a real relationship. She's decided, she said, to be gentle with both him and herself when there's tension between them, instead of dredging up the complaints of the past.

"We've wasted too many years struggling rather than loving each other," she told me recently. "Al and I have chosen not to whip ourselves over what we might have done differently or what we might have done wrong. We're in our seventies, and we don't want to lose any more precious time with our son by fretting over what might have been. We've chosen to forgive ourselves and accept that we misunderstood Tim and ourselves, but we have never stopped loving him and we've been working hard to love better. It took a while to get here, but I can honestly say we love him, trust his choices, and want whatever he decides is best for him. We did our best even when we didn't understand Tim very well. In fact, by going through all that we did to understand him, I think we came to a place of love and affection that we might not have found otherwise. Not to say it has been easy, but there was a blessing in it."

Stepping back to examine a long-standing conflict, you have a chance to reflect on your own behavior and to reconnect with the humanity of the complicated people lost inside that old battle. Forgiveness and love can often be the result.

Letting the Old Fights Go

As we look through our pasts for what needs forgiveness, one thing we discover again and again is that we're not the same as we were when an old grievance took root. We've grown, changed, developed—we're not the adolescents or even the adults we used to be. In reviewing old hurts, we frequently find that the sting is gone, or we can't quite remember what upset us so much. And in forgiving—or simply letting the conflict rest—we bring our sense of self into the present, whether that's a conscious process or it happens unconsciously as forgiveness takes place.

From this vantage point in life, we can see farther and deeper, which allows us to realize that holding onto old grievances has created a distance between us and others that has damaged our souls more than the original offense ever did. We feel an increasingly strong pull to clean things up, to feel good about ourselves as we try to answer: What kind of person am I really? What kind of life have I really had? How well have I loved?

Lynn, a member of one of my groups, told us how her family had been torn apart when she was in college and her brother joined a fundamentalist church. "We weren't religious at all, and it was a shock when Alan joined a faith that seemed to condemn anyone outside it. One side of our family is Jewish, and according to Alan's church, all of us were going straight to Hell. That offended me deeply, and I felt as though I couldn't see my brother inside the dogma. We had always been close, and I felt like he'd been snatched away. I was grief-stricken. And then I was angry. I hardly talked to him for years, in part because he seemed to reject his whole past—including me— and deliberately kept his distance. But as time passed, I realized that I had to admire what he made of his life and his own family. I don't agree with his church's positions about a lot of things, but they're generous to the poor, and they do community work that I respect. Even so, out of habit, I stayed away. I was afraid to bring up what I was thinking. I didn't want to get into another argument about not being born again."

Then, Lynn said, her father got sick, and in the months before he died she was talking to Alan on the phone every day, coordinating appointments or consultations with doctors. "I had been looking through old photos and found a photo-booth strip of the three of us, Dad with me and Alan on his lap, making faces and laughing, and I pulled it out to take on my next visit to the nursing home. I thought to myself, 'What happened to us?' I don't even care about Alan's religion anymore. I haven't cared much for a long time. I just wanted my brother, and I wanted to know his kids, too. We're all we've got. The next time I saw him, I apologized for my part in keeping us apart, and without saying anything about forgiveness, I privately forgave him for all those things I had held against him for so long. He put his arm around me and said, 'You know I love you, Sis.'

"I don't even remember if he made any apologies. I realized I didn't need any," she said. "We're not in our twenties and trying to change each other anymore. We are the only people who know our crazy family history, and that makes us particularly appreciate each other. We don't talk religion, but we can talk about our shared values and our growing-up years. We don't venture into politics, which is just fine. I think when Dad got sick and there was so much for us to take care of together, so many decisions to make, we saw that we have a core bond that's more important than who we each vote for or what he believes will happen to me after I die. I wish we could've gotten here sooner. I've been looking for other old grudges in my life that I want to say goodbye to," she told us. "One thing I know now that I didn't know then: Life is short, and love is precious. Much too precious to waste."

Death is never too far away once we enter later life, and our appreciation for the "core bonds" between us and those who've been important to us—even if they've been distant or estranged for a while—can be stronger now than long-standing hurts.

That was a lesson we reminded each other of repeatedly in our discussions of forgiveness. With Death and our Wise Self advising us, we have a chance to ask: How much do we want to cling to the story of a hurt instead of quietly letting it be, not forgotten, but not constantly fed? How much bigger are we than our pain? What would it cost us to forgive?

Beyond Regrets and Recrimination: What's the Rest of the Story?

When regrets over dreams abandoned or left undone burden us, forgiveness can be particularly freeing. From inside our minds, the punishing stories we may tell ourselves—that we're failures, that we're lazy, and we don't have what it takes—seem fair and justified, so familiar that we hardly notice their cruelty. The judgments ring true. The harsh criticism and attacks seem earned. We talk to ourselves in ways we'd never allow someone else to talk to a person we loved. And it can be tremendously healing to offer ourselves the gift of acceptance—*Yes, what happened is a part of my story that's brought me pain*—and forgiveness—*There's more to me and my story than that. I can let the pain and self-punishment go.* In learning to hold the space between those opposites, we can refocus and begin to see and breathe life into the hopeful, nuanced human who lives inside the cruel caricatures we've sometimes held of ourselves.

Carl, the computer analyst in our life-review group, had been full of self-recrimination as he talked about his failure to open the bookstore he had dreamed of, referring to himself as timid and gutless and a disappointment to himself and the people who believed in him. But what was the rest of the story? I suggested that he might try accessing it by writing a note to himself from his Wise Self, who could see a broader picture. What would a wise, kind friend say to make the story more complete? How would that friend comfort and encourage him? What gifts had his choices in the past given him that could feed his dream now?

Talking over what he might say, we came up with statements like: "Carl, you are a good person who did the best he could with what he had to work with at the time—including the present. You are a cautious, methodical man who has a talent for making well-considered choices about how to invest his time and energy. This talent takes the form of starting small and testing the situation to see how it goes." We began enumerating the steps Carl *had* taken toward his dream. "You've experimented in many ways, starting a book group at temple, researching what it might take to start your own store. Your steadiness has allowed you to put aside a nest egg that could help you launch a small business. Maybe you'll try a 'pop-up' somewhere to test the waters. Waiting until now to try has given you reserves and ideas and experience you didn't have before. Your desire is stronger than it's ever been."

And we spoke to the real sense of possibility Carl had always kept alive below the self-criticism: "Many successful people begin their heart's desire later in life, when they are actually more ready to move ahead with concrete plans. You are one of those people. You have been preparing yourself to take this risk. You've built the security you need and you have never let your dream die. You can trust yourself. Whatever you regret losing is already gone. But your dream is here, tugging at you as it has for so long. It believes in you. You are worth believing in. You are worthy of trust."

Carl was surprised at the forgiving, accepting words he found to describe his experience and said he was a little uncomfortable giving himself this "pep talk." But his mood lightened as we continued, especially when he quoted the words from his Wise Self: "You are worth believing in. You are worthy of trust." For as much as he had told himself the opposite, this was the large, embracing truth he longed to hear.

A Final Tool: Meditations to Open the Heart to Forgiveness

"We all did the best we could with what we knew at the time" can be used as a sort of healing mantra. The words resonate because we know we aren't the same people we were in the past. We didn't have the skills, experience, and insight that we have now. We've learned and grown, and our mistakes have brought us precious understandings about who we are. In seeing the layered truth about ourselves, and recognizing that the same mix of negative and positive, blundering and skill is also true of others, we've opened the door for compassion.

Now I think it's possible for us to open ourselves to some of the most soul-lifting words we can hear or say: "I forgive you"; "Please forgive me"; and "I forgive myself." We didn't begin here because often people think that saying "I forgive you" will automatically loosen the hold of deep hurts and grievances and disappointments. But to reduce the power of the emotions and expectations that have kept old hurts and grievances alive, we need to learn and choose new ways of understanding and responding. Doing that gives us more space to breathe, so we can come into the present and offer compassion to ourselves and others. We've been learning and practicing *acts* of forgiveness. That makes it easier, now, to let words of forgiveness penetrate the heart and heal the soul.

The forgiveness exercises below are based on the work of Jack Kornfield, whose books and video meditations on forgiveness offer wonderful support for this deep and liberating inner work. They're deceptively simple, with the power to ring through you and bring profound change. I'd like to leave you with these to close our work with forgiveness. I hope you'll return to them, and all the tools in this chapter, to bring yourself peace.

Meditation One: Seeking Forgiveness from Others
Settle yourself in a safe, quiet place where you won't be interrupted. Now close your eyes and take three deep, slow breaths, emphasizing the exhale. As your body and mind still, allow yourself to reflect on the ways you have harmed others over the course of your life, the

ways you have acted unskillfully and hurtfully out of confusion or fear or anger. Feel your sadness and regret over what you've done.

Now imagine that you are in an open green field, standing in front of one person you've harmed because of something you've done or failed to do. Look into that person's face. You have a chance right now to ask for forgiveness. Know that as you do, you can release the regret and pain you've carried so long. You can set that burden down. Look into the eyes of this person and remember how you hurt them. You've both been burdened by the hurt ever since. Feel your sorrow, your sincere remorse. When you're ready, say, "I ask for your forgiveness. Please forgive me." Repeat the words if you need to. "I ask for your forgiveness. Please forgive me. I ask for your forgiveness. Please forgive me." Embrace the other person from the heart, and when you're ready, let them disappear. If you want to summon other people, living or dead, into this field of forgiveness, do. There's no need to rush.

When you feel complete, take three deep, slow breaths and open your eyes. Notice any lightness you feel. Know that you can return to this place anytime you choose.

Meditation Two: Forgiving Those Who Have Hurt You

As before, settle yourself in a safe, quiet place and close your eyes. Take three deep, slow breaths. Now call to mind the many ways you have been injured by other's words or actions, or what they've failed to say or do. All of us have been abandoned, let down, and betrayed, knowingly or unknowingly. All of us have been hurt.

Remember the ways and times people have harmed you, acting unskillfully and hurtfully out of their own confusion, fear, anger, or pain. Feel the weight of any resentment, pain, and anger you still carry in your heart because of those actions. Know that it's in your power to gently release this pain. You don't need to feed it or hold it close anymore and continue to suffer. You can choose to let it be and turn to the present, as best you can. That is forgiveness.

Breathing and remembering, call to mind one person whose actions have hurt you and say, "I choose to feed the light inside me instead of the darkness. In the best way I can, I forgive you. I wish you peace." Repeat this several times: "In the best way I can, I forgive you. I wish you peace."

Notice how you feel. Be gentle with yourself if your heart is slow to catch up with your mind's desire to forgive. The words may just feel like words at first, but allow your heart to open little by little and the light inside yourself to connect with the light that may seem hidden inside the other person. Return to this exercise as you need to, as you feel the desire to forgive.

Meditation Three: Forgiving Yourself

Centering yourself and breathing deeply, close your eyes and call to mind your own face as a child, as a young person, as the person you are today. Remember the many ways you have caused yourself pain, acting with harshness or cruelty toward yourself, the times you have let yourself down. Feel the pain and sadness of the times you have betrayed yourself, abandoned yourself, struggled, failed. Know that you can release the burden of that pain. You did the best you could as the person you were then, years ago and yesterday. Know that as the person you are today, you can open your heart and feed the best of yourself with kindness, with gentleness, with love. Repeat to yourself: "I offer myself forgiveness for the many ways I've hurt myself out of confusion or fear or anger or pain. I gently release any regret or recrimination. I forgive myself. I forgive myself. I forgive myself."

CHAPTER SIX

THE SIXTH TASK

Look at the Past and Present
through the Lens of Gratitude

"If the only prayer you say in your whole life is thank you,
that would be enough."

MEISTER ECKHART

Reviewing your life sets you on course for the fresh start of your wisdom years. It gives you a chance to let go of fixed interpretations of who you and other people were, making way for what you can be. And, combined with forgiveness work, it lets you face what has hurt you and stood in your way so you can begin to clear it away.

A last key step in this process of shifting and updating your perspective on your past involves mining for gold in any parts of your life that still trouble you and looking for what was of value in the hard times and in situations that were full of pain. In that way you can try out a way of being that can bloom in later life, less quick to see things as black or white, more inclined and able to call on your heart to see what the ego and the head couldn't. What I'm talking about, though it may not sound like it, is looking through the lens of gratitude.

Leading gratitude researcher Robert Emmons defines gratitude as "an acknowledgment that we have received something of value from others," or, I'd add, from any situation we've experienced. Acknowledging the light inside the dark, the value of *everything* we've been through, these researchers tell us, can connect us with an awareness of the benevolence that runs through our lives. Just that sense, they say, can make us feel more positive, more resilient.

Gratitude begins with noticing that we have received a benefit that has come to us from outside ourselves, through the good intentions of another person or through other benevolent forces.

It's worth paying attention to the components that lead to gratitude because each one gives us a way to summon and understand it:

- The acknowledgment—*Yes, something good happened. Look, what a gift.*
- The fact that it came from outside us—*I didn't make this happen, will it, or earn it. Its source wasn't me.*
- The sense of benevolence—*What outside forces set in motion has an ultimate benefit for me.*

Viewing an event in this way draws us into an almost magical layer of the world that's always been just an acknowledgment away, a realm of gifts and appreciation that's entered through the open, thankful heart. When we look at our lives through the lens of gratitude, we see that strewn abundantly through the difficulties we've faced are moments that make us glad. (I like the word *glad* because its root meanings— bright, shining, joyous—capture what gratitude produces in us and allows us to see.) Ordinary life often reveals itself to be remarkable. A shining gift. A bright blessing. An occasion for joy.

It may seem frivolous, saccharine, or unrealistic to spend time searching out and appreciating the hidden gifts in our lives, but it's actually highly practical. Practicing gratitude has been found to help people cope with stress and loss and increase their levels of happiness and sense of satisfaction with their lives. Studies have found that it reduces inflammation in heart patients and speeds their recovery; lessens depression; strengthens social bonds; and helps people cultivate wisdom, humility, and patience.

I know from personal experience that it lifts and soothes the soul.

We can cultivate an expansive gratitude that values all of our experiences and makes every part of our lives, even our suffering, sacred. As we make this way of seeing a practice, then a habit of the heart, we draw ever closer to our Wise Self, closer to joy, closer to the sense of wonder at the core of us. Gratitude can come as we cherish the brilliance of a flower in a shaft of sun and as we look back at the way our resilient heart came through a crushing loss. It can come as we cherish the sweet and bitter, the ordinary we no longer take for granted, the light that sparks in our darkest times. We can become thankful for the gift of it all.

Seeing the Webs of Connection

Gratitude comes more easily in later life as the ego eases its grip, and we can finally stop clinging to the narrative that says: "I did it myself. I worked hard, overcame the odds, and I earned my way to where I am." When we look more closely at our stories of independence and solo accomplishment, we often find that they're threads of a rich tapestry of *inter*dependence: Through it all, the "I" that accomplished so much and did the hard work of becoming had the generous help of others. Much of the goodness that flows through our lives, we find, didn't come to us because we sought it or earned it or deserved it. It was a gift.

Frederick Streng, a comparative religions scholar, writes that as "people recognize that they are connected to each other in a mysterious and miraculous way" they sense that much of the good in their lives occurs because they're "part of a wider, or transcendent context."

It can be inspiring, humbling, and even awe-inspiring to take note of the times that we've experienced "mysterious and miraculous" connections to helping hands and blessings that have come to us unbidden. It's impossible to remember those times without gratitude.

As I reviewed my past, I was surprised to see how often I had entered a current of benevolence without realizing it, meeting strangers who said encouraging words at just the right moment, or crossing paths with those whose kindness and generosity changed the course of my life. I've been rescued, uplifted, guided, and loved by people (and creatures) who offered what I needed most—often before I knew I needed it. I used to tell myself that when things turned out well, it was the result of my own effort, talents, and resourcefulness. But more often than not, as I looked back, I saw that kind hands had guided me along, opening my way, enlarging my sense of what was possible.

One unexpected benefactor arrived when I was in my thirties and in the midst of work that had consumed me for many years: sitting at the bedsides of dying cancer patients and using what I learned there to train volunteers to help them. It was intense and gratifying, but living so close to so much loss for so long took an emotional toll.

I met my benefactor, the husband of one of the volunteers, after giving a talk about how the patients who survived cancer often seemed to have faith in something larger than themselves. Many survivors I'd talked to told me that they had a mission in life to complete, and it had struck me that they were much like businesspeople I'd met who were able to pull off daunting, "impossible" projects—like sending men to the moon—because of their strong belief in their mission. I labeled them all *Peak Performers*.

The volunteer's husband, a senior executive at IBM, lit up when he heard my "peak performance" idea and invited me to speak to a conference of his corporate managers. When they responded enthusiastically, he invited me back to coach his team on applying the concept to their day-to-day operations. He also submitted my name to several speakers' bureaus, describing me as an "expert on peak performance"—a label I'd never have given myself.

My phone began to ring, and suddenly I really was a peak performance expert, and an opportunity for a change I hadn't known I needed opened up before me. I was excited and energized by talking about life instead of death, and I realized that now I could spend my days doing just that.

It seemed, and still seems, astonishing to me that the man heard my talk, and then stepped in to help me shift course. Essentially, he invented a new career for me, put me on a rocket, and lit the fuse. You'd think he was a close friend or mentor, but I hardly knew him. And I have nothing but gratitude for his kindness to me.

When I think about this man I wonder: What would have happened if he had not been in the audience? My mind and ego tell me I would've been fine. But what would I have done had this man not guided me onto a new track? Would I have kept pushing myself at the hospital and wound up with compassion fatigue and burnout? Would I have been able to admit to myself that a part of my life was over? Would I ever have had the kinds of experiences that came when people embraced the idea of peak performance? I can't know, but I am certain that because of one man's kindness, my life changed dramatically for the better. And my gratitude for that is off the charts.

The question: "What might've been different if X had not happened?" is a powerful tool for highlighting the impact of benevolent actions, people, and happenstances. Gratitude researchers call this "mental subtraction," and they've found it to be a highly effective way of cultivating gratitude as we see how much of the goodness in our lives is shaped not by our will and efforts and plans, but by chance, generosity, and the grace of something outside us.

Look back through the stories of joy or accomplishment in your life and try tracing the circumstances, the interventions of others, and those "gifts" that had to come together to make possible what happened. For all your careful planning and hard work, what outside factors converged to give you reasons for gratitude?

Practice: The Gratitude Journal

Gratitude is easy to access when we look at the joyful surprises of life, and it's good to start there in making gratitude a habit of the heart. Simply noticing kind acts, happy accidents, moments of beauty, and unexpected reasons for relief or thanks amplifies our awareness of the currents of benevolence that are always carrying us. It becomes harder to take for granted the gifts that fill a day, or a life.

Robert Emmons and other gratitude researchers suggest expanding our capacity for this kind of noticing with gratitude lists, a tool that escaped from their studies into pop culture with a significant boost from Oprah. You may have discounted such lists as gimmicky or superficial, but I highly recommend this simple practice.

Emmons advises stopping once or twice a week to look back at what happened and write down five things for which you're thankful.

It's most meaningful and powerful, he says, to use specific details to briefly describe the particulars that made the event or action or experience feel like a gift. It's also helpful to make a point of remembering the positive events that *surprised* you. Doing that will help keep you awake to—and, if you're like me, constantly struck by—the endless variety of goodness that flows through your life.

Pay attention to the circumstances that heighten your feelings of gratitude, for instance, knowing that the situation bringing you so much happiness (a vacation, a beautiful stroll in the country) will end soon or that your time with someone you love is short, both of which heighten the desire to savor and appreciate every moment.

In scanning your life for gifts and blessings, you might incorporate the concept of *firgun*, a modern Hebrew term that refers to finding joy and gratitude in someone else's good fortune, something I feel increasingly as time goes on. You might also pay attention to the intense feeling of thanks and relief that comes with hearing good news after you've feared the worst for yourself or someone else. There is power, too, in letting Death sit near you, reminding you that you are here now to soak in the colors of sunrise, but you won't always be. That poignant knowing makes our experience all the more sweet.

Notice it all, and fill your lists with vivid, varied reasons for thanks.

Keeping these lists in a gratitude journal allows you to look back across time to see a steady stream of positive moments, kindnesses, and gifts—from people or nature or the Universe—that you can savor each time you think of them. Recalling them in detail (the reason to note specifics on your list) keeps them alive, and it will make you ever more attentive to the richness of what you're receiving, or have received.

Emmons says that "gratitude fatigue" often sets in when people try to keep a daily gratitude list. He and other researchers have noticed that we adapt rapidly to positive events when we start focusing on them, and no longer feel the happiness boost that comes when we make this practice more regular, and perhaps more rote. So it's good to set a regular time to stop, just a couple of times a week, and bring your full attention back to the act of appreciation and thanks.

In recording the small things—the way a stranger's smile and comments in a checkout line lifted your spirits, the joy an unexpected postcard brought, the way blazing reds and purples of a sky filled your heart, the pleasure of stroking a loved one's cheek—we shake ourselves awake to the wonder of the ongoing goodness in life.

Using Gratitude to Ease Our Way through Time and Change
I've been fascinated by the way that feeling gratitude in the moment changes not only the moment, but also our relationship with past and future. It eases our way through time.

At seventy-five, I can't pretend that challenges and unwelcome change don't come thick and fast at times. Friends call with news of surgery, and death keeps shrinking my circle of dear ones. Doctors' visits become an ever-larger part of all our routines, and the list of watched and worrisome conditions lengthens. Familiar touchstones of the past disappear—"small" things, like a beloved store or corner tree or the elderly dry cleaner whose smile was something you could count on every time you came in. Even the seasons can seem wrong— too hot or dry or cold, the very air unfamiliar, not like before. Not like before.

In later life, we can string these changes and erasures and concerns into a litany of loss, a constant state of mourning and complaint and irritation. But gratitude opens us to a way of navigating change that is expansive, uplifting, joyful.

When you look at the past with an appreciation of what you've loved and gratitude for the time you shared, you carry the spark of that love into the present, where it can walk in the world with you, inspire you, and keep you company instead of taunting you with a sense of diminishment and loss.

I was at dinner with a longtime friend when his knee locked as he stood to go to the men's room. He grimaced and eased himself up, then slowly limped away. He was grumbling when he returned—*damn knee*—and I knew that our conversation could easily turn into an organ recital—his knee, my hip, and our shared medley of pains and the procedures to fix them. But I wondered what it would be like to put all that aside. "Here's a question for you," I said. "What do you remember most about the times it served you well? You were quite a hiker weren't you?"

"I was a hiker, and you were Pocket Hercules," he said with a laugh.

We started talking about what it had felt like to be strong young men and throw ourselves into joys that let us revel in our bodies. We stood back and admired those earlier versions of ourselves. We cringed a little, too. Those younger selves were competitive and certain of their immortality, yet also insecure, hiding their vulnerability behind an armor of muscles and proving their fearlessness by pushing their bodies hard. They'd rest when they were dead, they said. "We were a couple of lunkheads sometimes," my friend said with obvious affection. Our earlier antics had put a lot of wear and tear on us, but there was nothing to regret. We stood next to the athletes we'd been, savoring their youth and feeling their raw energy. It was all there in sense memory and twined into our spirits, there to appreciate and enjoy.

That's true of the people and places and tastes we've loved, the songs and stories. We keep them alive in us by recalling them not with nostalgic longing but with thanks.

Using Gratitude to Find the Light Inside Dark Times

I've found that in life-review work, gratitude can be a vehicle and tool for looking again at the dark times we've experienced and finding a reason for thanks or appreciation even for what hurt us the most. In my life and in the lives of many people I've known, I've seen that some of the most important openings and growth have come from experiences that could be looked upon as reversals, losses, tragedies, or plain bad luck.

It's not a matter of slapping on a smile and saying "make lemonade" or "look on the sunny side." I would never ask anyone to do that. But I've found it revealing and productive to ask:

- Who am I now that I never would've been without having to face the experiences that most challenged me?
- Who or what showed me the way when I was lost or lifted me up when I felt defeated?
- What did they teach me?
- Might there be lessons and discoveries about my deeper self that I can carry forward now?
- How does my suffering connect me to those who also suffer in this world?
- And what have my most difficult experiences taught me of grace?

This is challenging work, but it eases the way for forgiveness, acceptance, and even joy.

Bharat, a sixty-year-old friend who works as a counselor, has been shaped by a life strewn with obstacles. Born to teenage parents, he was abandoned by his father when he was a baby. He grew up searching and feeling hopeless about the future, and he was shaken to learn at thirteen that he had been adopted. "I always felt like a fatherless child," he told me. "I had no real father figure, especially no support emotionally." For many years he had felt pained, even haunted, by his father's absence, wondering what kind of person could have set a baby boy adrift without protection.

But when he talks about the wound of being abandoned, he never fails to think about what saved him, a stream of men who nurtured a sustaining element of his life, his spirituality. "In my teens and twenties, I had several mentors who took me under their wings and helped me with the problems I'd been having with my family," he said. "They showed me a radically different perspective on life, a way of thinking psychologically about my very troubled family." At eighteen, he met his first spiritual teacher and mentor, who introduced him to the Ram Dass book *Be Here Now*. "It gave me purpose," he says. Then a college professor and mentor led him to the works of Carlos Castaneda and Chogyam Trungpa Rinpoche, the Tibetan Buddhist teacher. And through that professor, Bharat, then twenty, met Ram Dass.

"My mentors changed my whole outlook and purpose in life," he said. "They saw a worthwhile person in me. They are why I went to college and cultivated my spiritual nature, my commitment to self-development through service."

He was tested mightily in his late twenties when he contracted HIV. Living with the virus has been a tremendous challenge, with many physical and emotional ups and downs. It would be easy for Bharat to focus on the difficult elements of his life and see himself as first abandoned, then knocked down by disease just as he began to come into his own. But perhaps because his life was so precarious during the early years of his illness, Bharat has a long and deep habit of gratitude, going back to the period when surviving another day, and then a day after that, was a reason for celebration. Gratitude—for doctors and friends and spiritual comfort, for caretakers and teachers, for the next new drug, the next day of life, the next breath—was a means of transcending despair. It's our ability to cultivate such a perspective that brings us resilience, peace, even joy as we travel through our own times of doubt, testing, and fear.

"Now that I'm sixty, it drives home the reality that I've been living for thirty-two years with HIV, which was initially a one- to two-year prognosis," he says. "I've lived over thirty years more than what was expected and, for that, I have tremendous gratitude.

"I'm human," he adds. "I've sometimes felt it was unfair that this happened to me and wished that things had gone another way. But some of the greatest gifts of my life have come from living with this disease. I connect with my clients and have more to give them because I have felt the kind of pain they're going through. And so many people have helped me, even strangers who've shown me how much I am loved." Does that make HIV a wonderful thing? Of course not. Would he have much preferred perfect health and a chance to know a loving father? Absolutely. But we don't get to take away the painful parts of our histories. We don't have that choice. All we can control is the way we interpret what happened.

As he looked back at his childhood from the age of sixty, Bharat found a new and healing path to gratitude. He felt the familiar ache of being abandoned by his father. But now he could imagine his father as the same kind of confused boy-man he'd been at eighteen, before he met his first mentor: drifting, starved for loving guidance, angry at his fate, afraid. His heart opened to the man he'd never known. The pain of that early loss has softened into an appreciation for the accident of fate that pushed his father and mother together just long enough to bring him into being. He felt a deep gratitude for that.

It's often said that forgiveness and gratitude are twin flames, with one igniting the other to illuminate and expand our understanding of what we've been through. As we practice the actions that allow us to forgive and accept others and our circumstances, a sense of gratitude often seems to overtake us. It's natural for the work you've done and are doing with forgiveness to spill over into thanks.

Letting Gratitude Ease Regret

Gratitude was an unexpectedly useful tool when members of our life-review group had trouble forgiving themselves for choices they had made and for staying in ill-fitting situations that they looked back on as a waste of precious life. All of us had made mistakes, persisted on paths we knew were wrong for us or hurt someone else, and even with the intellectual understanding that everyone involved had done the best we could with what we knew, it was sometimes hard to shake the regret and self-recrimination.

Chip had chosen a safe marriage with a woman who needed him and "would never leave me." From the time they were engaged, he told us, he'd heard a voice in his head that said, "Don't do it! She's not right for you. You'll end up trapped in a loveless marriage." But Chip married Glenda anyway. He spent fifteen years struggling with the feeling that he'd made a terrible mistake, and he was shocked but relieved when Glenda solved the problem a couple of years ago by leaving him for somebody else.

"I've been trying to forgive myself for staying all those years and doing all that rationalizing," he said. "I told myself that at least we were together and doing okay financially and at work. What we had wasn't any worse than a lot of other marriages I saw. It was better than what my parents had after they broke up. But it was wrong for me, wrong for her. I'll never get those years back, and neither will she."

He decided to ask the wise part of himself, "How can I get over this regret and forgive myself for being such an idiot for so long?" He told us he'd write letters to himself—*Dear Chip* letters, he called them—to "hold the relationship up to the light" and see if he could see new facets, something that would redeem the experience for him somehow.

I suggested that he might jumpstart the letters with questions that could help him unearth insights he'd gained through his marriage and breakup, "gifts" of the experience he could draw on in the future. Some of the questions are based on Emmons's gratitude work, and I've found them to be valuable in helping me—and many others—find wisdom in our wounds.

In Chip's letters, he asked himself:

- What did you learn about yourself, positive and negative, from the situation?
- What did you learn about yourself in dealing with the situation/its aftermath that surprised you? What strengths did it draw from you?
- In what ways did the pain or struggle make you more the person you want to be?

Chip also thought about what he most wanted in his next partners and relationships.

He told us that the ache and anger he'd felt toward himself eased as he looked back on the marriage and reflected on what he'd learned. "I thought back to the beginning, when I was so relieved to find someone who would never leave me. Glenda wasn't a compromise for me, she was exactly what I wanted, a partner who was loyal above everything else. I had forgotten about that. After I saw my parents' bad divorce, I wanted someone who would stay forever. Back then I wanted security more than I wanted sex, which is saying something. That's how I could keep talking myself into staying. But in my gut, I always knew that what I really wanted was someone who wanted me for me, not someone who stayed because she was too scared to be on her own. I get that now.

"The past couple of years have taught me that I can stand to be alone. I realized that since Glenda left me, I've been able to 'divorce' the part of myself that was so afraid I couldn't survive on my own or live through a breakup. I'm stronger than I thought. If something doesn't work out, I'll be okay. I can take chances now that I was too afraid to take back then. I want to listen to my gut, and I want to find love. I think I can.

"I don't wish Glenda anything but good," he said. "We gave each other what we could, and thank god she finally ended it. Now we're both free to have the love we wanted all along. We went through a lot together, and it wasn't *all* bad. She was there for me when I was sick and when my folks were struggling, and she was always kind. She's a good person. We were totally wrong for each other, but we tried. The divorce hit me hard, but I'm proud of the way I got through it."

Chip decided to enter a therapy group for divorced people where he could explore what he was learning from the letters. Currently, he's dating one of the women he met there. "She is very different than

Glenda," he told me. "She's strong and independent, but at the same time, she's so loving. I feel lucky to know how right she is for me."

Gratitude for Mistakes, Our Great Teachers

We learn who we are, and become who we're meant to be, by trying and failing, seeing what works, what doesn't. And in the process, we pick up skills and compassion and a sense of what truly suits us. We learn by listening to those whispers of wisdom that come in gut feelings and clear-sighted moments that tell us something's amiss. And sometimes instead of paying attention, we blow it. We simply don't get things right the first time around, especially as we grow, and "what's right for us" evolves into something strange and new.

John O'Donohue, the wonderful Irish writer, considered our mistakes to be the most precious moments on our soulful journey through life. And seen that way, they are gifts.

Gratitude and forgiveness come, I have learned, when we realize that everything we've done in this lifetime has contributed to who we are now. Everything has been a teacher—including the missteps and wounds—and through it all, we've unexpectedly grown.

Like Chip, I had a long marriage that felt right at the beginning and empty by the end. I could strongly relate to his feelings of regret—I'd had them too. But a few years back when I came across some photos from that time and showed them to my wife Cindy, she suggested that I see my ex and give her copies of the pictures. After thirty years of having no contact at all, we met for lunch, two people who had once been young and uneasily married, and we looked at the photo albums I'd brought.

"Oh, we were so innocent," my ex-wife said.

"It's okay if you really want to say 'so dumb,'" I said.

She laughed. "That too. Dumb isn't quite fair, though. There was so much we didn't know."

Sitting there, it was clear to us both that we were incredibly different, and I wished I could have seen that as a kid. I understood from the vantage point of my seventies that our relationship could never have succeeded because we weren't that compatible. Yet for all the ways we were mismatched, we still shaped each other, learned together, in the dozen years we shared our lives. I'm a part of her, and she's a part of me. And perhaps because of her, I became clear about what I really did want in a partner, so when Cindy came along, I recognized her and knew immediately I wanted to get closer. I'm grateful for that. There's nothing now to regret or forgive in what came before. What lingers is gratitude.

Taking a moment to express feelings like that, out loud or by letter, can transform the past, infusing it with the peace that comes with the understandings of later life.

The shift from anger or impatience or resentment to gratitude starts, I believe, when we realize that we are learning something valuable from the situation and can honestly say, *Thank You*. That doesn't mean you don't hurt or that you forget the transgressions or pain or shortcomings, but rather that any situation or person can be a teacher. A sense of gratitude for that may develop over time—even years later—upon further reflection.

Transformed in this way, our wounds become our wisdom, and our pain becomes sacred.

Three Exercises for Carrying Gratitude across the Threshold into Your Wisdom Years

As we prepare to leave this chrysalis of life review and reflection, I'd like to suggest three ways you might carry the lessons and skills and especially the *energy* of gratitude into the decision-making and experiments that will shape your wisdom years.

EXERCISE 1:

Write a gratitude letter to someone, and share it with them in a gratitude visit.

The wonder, delight, and awe you feel at remembering how people have helped you is a gift you can share. In telling the givers how their action changed you, and what their help has meant in your life, you'll be letting them know in the most direct way possible that they've had a positive impact—not only on you but on the world you're connected to.

Share your happiness, your thanks. Emmons and other gratitude researchers suggest writing a heartfelt, one-page letter of thanks, and laminating it so you can present it and leave it behind. Meeting face-to-face lets you communicate your appreciation and warmth through your voice and body, not just your words, and it can let you both say what can only be said with laughter or tears or a hug.

You might surprise someone who perhaps unknowingly helped guide you toward a cherished goal. Or you might express the new gratitude you feel toward "difficult" people in your lives. In our life-review group, several members wrote gratitude letters to their Depression-era parents, offering warm thanks for the sacrifices they'd made to give their families the security that was so precious to them. You might also read aloud a gratitude letter to a person who's passed, which can enhance your appreciation of them.

If you'd like to go on a life-changing rampage of gratitude, make a list of the most significant people in your life and arrange gratitude visits to see and offer thanks to some or all of them. Researchers tell us that the sense of happiness and well-being that gratitude letters and visits produce can last for months and months and spur more acts of gratitude and generosity on both sides.

Some of the most resonant, powerful words you can tell anyone are: *Thank you. You changed my life. You made a difference.*

EXERCISE 2:
Look closely at your own stories of giving to discover
what you have received.

Like many people who have been drawn to a path of service in their lives, I'm deeply grateful anytime I'm able to do something to make someone's life better. It makes me feel good to help. But in reviewing my life lately, I've felt my gratitude deepening as I see how many vital, healing gifts have been offered to me by people I thought I was helping. I'm awed by our interconnectedness, and I think you may find the same is true as you think about similar instances in your life.

One of the most important people in my life is a young man named Jesse, whom I met when he was just ten years old. One version of our story is that a friend of mine knew Jesse, thought we might like each other, and invited me to a community center where he liked to play ball. My friend said Jesse was a "really bright, very athletic" kid, and she saw me as a likely mentor for him. Jesse had tremendous potential, I soon learned, but he hadn't had a lot of advantages in life. His East Oakland neighborhood was gang turf, and he didn't have a strong father figure at home. Sometimes there wasn't enough food or stimulation to nourish his fast-growing body and mind. He was a young black man in a city and a country suspicious of young black men.

We liked each other, and I got the idea that I could teach him my secrets to success. Jesse began spending weekends and holidays with Cindy and me at our Oakland Hills home, where he had his own bedroom and bathroom, a full refrigerator and, though I know it was trying for him at times, "non-stop access" to my lessons on positive values and achievement. Little by little, we got to know each other. I came to think of him as the son I never had, and to this day I call him my godson. Cindy and I took him to the Grand Canyon, encouraged him through his early dreams of becoming a football star or sports broadcaster, and proudly watched as he made the football squad and the Dean's List at Diablo Valley Community College. We suffered with him, too, as a torn ACL crushed his hopes. The pain and fear and doubt were intense, but he'd always talked about "helping kids from backgrounds like mine," and as his disappointment slowly healed, we reminded him of that calling and let him know we believed he had it in him to make it in college. Today, he's thriving as the headmaster of a private school—and he's the father of a new baby.

It's easy to revel in stories like that, which remind us of the way we can be a force for the good, large or small, in someone's life. But it's the story inside that story that my life review helped me appreciate— the story of what Jesse gave me.

When I met Jesse, I was a workaholic, constantly on the road with lectures and workshops, and only just beginning to sense that my bottomless drive was suffocating me. When a bright young man appeared in my life and needed my attention and love, it was as though my heart had called him in to save me. Jesse gave me a reason to be sure I spent more time at home and took breaks from travel. Something shifted in me as I realized that more than any lessons I wanted to teach him, what Jesse most needed from me was love and my steady presence in his life.

Six months after Jesse and I found each other, my father was diagnosed with cancer and given just a few months to live. As I sat with my dad, reviewing our complicated relationship, the time I'd spent fathering Jesse let me see Dad in a new light. My mom had always complained that my dad was a failure who'd never made it in life. She thought I needed a father who was as driven as she was. But at my core, I'd been much like Jesse, a smart kid who was hungry for love that didn't hinge on how well I competed. I was always trying to prove myself, and I craved the love of someone whose face lit up just to see me and never asked me to earn that love. Fortunately, I had that someone—Dad—but I'd never been able to see it. I thought fathers were supposed to be more like what my mom wanted, successful guys who gave you pep talks.

It was only because of my time with Jesse that I could finally feel the value of what Dad had given me. I'm deeply grateful that it happened while he was still alive, as it allowed me to let him know how much his love meant to me.

I thought that fate had brought Jesse and me together so I could help a disadvantaged boy, but now I can see that he was there to help *me* in a way that no one else could. He was the perfect person, appearing at the perfect time, to teach me about a father's love and help me understand all my father had given. I saw myself in Jesse, and I could see my father as though through Jesse's eyes.

Jesse became a catalyst who helped me rebalance my life and turn my focus from work to love. When Dad died, I can't say that I grieved less because Jesse was there—after all, Jesse had made me fully aware of what I was losing. But the boy who'd taught me so much about love and fathering and how much an old guy and a ten-year-old can be to each other, helped me keep my heart open and carry the best of my father into the world, gifts for which I will always be in his debt.

Question for reflection: Might there be places in your life where the "person you rescued" rescued you? What lessons about giving and gratitude might you take from that? What would it be like to tell that person with a gratitude letter and visit?

EXERCISE 3:

Write a declaration of thanks for the person you now see shining through the story of your life.

Finally, consider expressing your gratitude for the person you now see as you stand in later life looking back on all that's shaped you, helped you, and brought you to this moment. Write a letter, or a manifesto, describing who you are now. How are you different? What do you appreciate about yourself and your life that you didn't before?

Who does your Wise Self tell you that you are?

I'd like to share a declaration that my wife Cindy Spring wrote. Yours may be quite different, but I hope you'll tap the same energy of acceptance, forgiveness, gratitude, and excitement as you stand poised to embrace your wisdom years:

Cindy's Declaration of Self

I can see how all the things I've done in this lifetime have contributed to who I am now. How grateful I am to myself for my good choices, and how grateful I am to myself for all the errors that have given me such insights.

Who I am: A woman with a large, loving heart who cares about so many people, plants, and other species; who holds them in delight and in compassion and nurturance as well as she can. I am a human who in this incarnation has been given/has created the circumstances and the gifts to make contributions in many arenas—media, books, social justice, the environment, and now to the newly emerging spirituality.

As one of many midwives, I see it as much more expansive, inclusive, experiential, loving-without-judgment, and open-ended than anything I've ever known.

I am a person so incredibly blessed with a soul mate who is not only a perfect fit, but who *is* me and I am him. Two pieces that fit together to make a whole, a microcosm of the One.

I am a person blessed with so many friends who I love and cherish, and who love me.

I am Rita (my mother) at her best, with some of her foibles, too. We are finding each other again and helping each other to evolve even more. [She died in 1999.]

I am now someone who isn't afraid to be who she is. I don't have to project an ideal Cindy Spring. This has been evolving for some time now. I will continue to hone the crystal of who I am, polishing off the rough edges, learning how to love and laugh and counsel and teach and learn, and give with joy and abandon. May it be so.

PART THREE

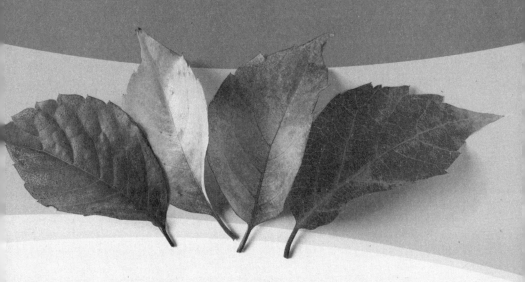

Opening

TO THE

Eternal

CHAPTER SEVEN

THE SEVENTH TASK

Using Your Gifts to
Nurture What Will Live On

"Now I become myself," May Sarton wrote of the stirred, shaken, reconfigured self we bring to later life. Now, with a clearer sense of who you've been, how your choices have shaped you, and what's at your core, it's possible to embrace the freedom of being fully yourself in later life and then in old age. You can insist on living from the soul out. Joseph Campbell is talking about exactly this when he speaks of giving ourselves over to the "rapture of being alive," filling our days with what we value most and doing what genuinely brings us bliss.

What would it look like to seed the world with the best of what you've become, to nourish what will outlive you, to do what you know now matters above all else?

To find out is to create your legacy as you home toward your own true north.

The ordinary demands of living don't disappear as we do this—there are still dishes to be done, errands to run, loved ones to tend, bills to pay, doctors' appointments to manage. But within the confines of everyday life, we can choose to nourish the extraordinary truth of who we are—and experience what happens when we bring our deepest loves more fully into our lives and the world.

Some of us have been waiting years or decades to do that. Some of us have put almost everything else ahead of what we've always known is most important and most central to who we are and want to be. But now it can—and should—be difficult to let that pattern of postponement continue. Especially because you've been actively challenging the tendency to delay your "real life" till later. Through our work so far, you've been exploring what brings you joy, and noticing the themes, passions, and gifts that have called to you again and again, and you're likely to feel them demanding your attention as you emerge from the chrysalis of reflection.

The manifesto you wrote to end the last chapter is a bold statement of who you've become. Now it's time to embrace it all.

Later life, as I've been saying, isn't simply a continuation of adult desires and priorities. Adulthood ends, just as adolescence ends. And something *new* takes its place. Not just decline, pain, and loss—though inevitably those come—but also this rapturous opportunity to do what feeds our soul. There's an urgency and sense of possibility that come with realizing we can, and must, live from the center in the time we have left. We don't have to carry on in "adult drag," pretending to be and want what we once were. Freedom comes in knowing we're different now, feeling what beckons from the heart in later life, and giving ourselves over to it.

This is the countdown. Who will you let yourself be?

Small Steps toward Larger Shifts

As I talked with my friend Lynn about this shift, she smiled and told me her life review had left her thinking about the summer between ninth and tenth grade, when she'd spent endless afternoons in her room thinking about the shy and awkward girl she'd been, and imagining who she wanted to become. "I was a little startled to remember how intentional I'd been about it," she said. "It wasn't that I had a romantic fantasy about the popular kids seeing me on the first day of school and saying, 'We never noticed how fun and interesting you are—come be our best friend.' It was me telling myself, 'I'm different now. I don't feel like that shy girl anymore. I'm not going to be her when I go back.'

"When you mentioned the idea of 'coming out of the chrysalis' in our sixties and seventies, I recognized that same feeling coming up in me," she said.

Lynn isn't planning to drop everything to reinvent herself. She's still working at age sixty-seven, and with no pension or significant savings to fall back on, she hopes to continue through her seventies if she can. But at the same time, she says she's determined not to simply carry on as before, and she's thinking more about the larger imprint she wants her life to leave.

"I'm truly not the same person I was when I stepped into this career. It's not just that I'm physically older. I'm at the point where I want to be sure the work adds up to something I believe in. I've spent a lot of my life thinking about making a living—and being grateful that I can. In marketing, I help people get their message across. I'm good at it, and it's satisfying. But lately it feels especially important for me to work for people and causes I believe in, to help the good guys who are in some way helping humanity and the planet. I had this idea of looking at the projects I work on from here on out as chapters of an ongoing story about how people can do good or thrive," she said.

"That doesn't seem like a big shift, but it is—knowing what's right work and what isn't. What fits in the story I want my life to tell. No matter what the job, I'd like to be someone who helps people talk about mutual respect and valuing the Earth and creating community—that's so much on my mind now, and I can move it more to the center of what I do."

It is liberating to look back to our beginnings, or even the self of ten years ago, and realize, "I'm not that version of myself anymore. I'm different." It's more liberating still to take even the smallest step, philosophical or physical, toward making the form and content of your life match who you are now. If you're still on the job, you might change the emphasis of your work, as Lynn is doing, or see what happens when you frame it in terms of legacy. What will you do differently, knowing that the fruits of *this moment* and the next are what you'll leave behind?

As Within, so Without—Changing Your Environment

On a simple level, you might decide to look closely at your physical surroundings and see how well the exterior of your life matches who you are now. Downsizing, a ritual for many of us in the wisdom years, often becomes the catalyst for a broader evaluation of what belongs with us in the future we envision for ourselves, and what no longer serves.

When my wife and I moved to a smaller place around the time I turned seventy, we shed many things we'd held onto for decades—books, trinkets from trips, clothes, furniture. It felt cathartic to lighten our load, both physically and emotionally. Once I was free of possessions I no longer related to, my new unburdened surroundings became a blank canvas for a kind of creative blossoming. The muse shows up more often, I find, when there's more room.

That was certainly true for Lynn.

"I think everything is more up for grabs now," she told me. "We thought we might need to move out of our apartment recently, and that prompted me to go through years of accumulated stuff to see if I was holding onto things that didn't really mean anything to me. It was quite the project. I gave away twenty bags of books, some from college, along with heaps of clothing and souvenirs from what seemed like someone else's life.

"What remains now is *chosen*," she said. "The whole process got us talking about how we really want to live. We were joking about a commune—you might laugh, but it got me interested in checking out some new possibilities. I'm looking at co-housing, where there's an intentional community of mixed ages, and everyone participates in decision-making and meeting the community's needs. You might help with gardening, and I might help a neighbor's kids with homework or put together a newsletter. And maybe we'd share the vacuum cleaner. I thought we might give it a try. It speaks to my heart, the idea of that kind of extended and chosen family. I think it suits my nature; Michael's too. So why not? That seems to be my new mantra: 'Why not?'"

EXERCISE:

Look Around. Does Your Home Feel Like You?

Don't underestimate the power of context as you imagine the possibilities of later life. Your environment and surroundings have a powerful influence on your awareness, motivation, and emotional state, and stirring them up often sends new impulses through your psyche.

As you look around the place you live, do you see a reflection of your current self? If not, make a conscious choice to rectify that during this transition to the wisdom years. What "looks like you?" What no longer belongs? What spaces can you open up for the muse?

What Will *Your* Later Life Story Be?

Inside the seemingly smaller questions of what to keep and what to give away, larger ones loom: How then *shall* we live, knowing better now who we are? What sort of legacy do we hope to leave, as the result of this life, and what steps will lead us toward that end?

I can't tell you what to do with the rest of your life. But I can help you feel your way toward it. This is different, as you've undoubtedly noticed, from "retirement planning," which often assumes that filling up the day is an end in itself. The goal of planning a life that reflects who you are in your wisdom years is to fill your days with *meaning*.

I often suggest that people focus on what I call legacy projects as a way of pivoting toward what will bring the most fulfillment. Legacy projects are ideas and undertakings that capture our imagination and give outward expression to the parts of ourselves we care most about and want to share. As you'll see, these projects are as varied as we are. They may reflect dormant talents or dreams that can finally bloom in the spaciousness that replaces working life. But they may also be unexpected responses to impulses that overtake us or desires that reveal themselves gradually, an inkling or workshop or experiment at a time.

At this stage, we live with what the poet David Whyte calls an "intimacy with disappearance," and the undeniable reality that we, too, will disappear. Against that backdrop, we're compelled to ask again and again: "What would I like to leave to the world that enriches it when I'm gone?" Our answers may lead us to tell our stories; create meaning and beauty through craft or art or works of imagination; and find opportunities to offer our company, counsel, and comfort to others. Some of us want to build organizations, set up charities, join movements. Many more of us will find our legacy work woven into the intimate realms of our lives, in the art we make of our gardens and friendships and family time.

The shift toward wisdom in later life is a shift toward spiritual and moral values like beauty, compassion, justice, or joy that are expressions of our higher self and the potential we all have available to us. So pay particular attention to the values you see as most important now. In these years, we become clearer and clearer about what remains as family goes, friends go, the body goes: It's the beauty and compassion and joy and love we share.

This clarity begets new priorities, releases new or old passions, becomes the expression of our wise, or wiser, soul. When people talk about legacy and feel "just right" about their choice of a legacy project, it's most often because they've found a way to concretely express one or more of their higher values.

You'll know a legacy project is right for you by the joy that it brings, the excitement that comes in doing or even thinking about it, and a sense that the opportunity to spend time this way is a blessing, not an obligation. It's a chance to lose yourself in a kind of aliveness that will resonate through time.

Whatever you choose, do it for love.

EXERCISE:

Gather Legacy Images

A good way to step into the question of legacy is to scan your life review for insights about the values that rise to the top for you now, and then consider how you might honor them. Let your intuition guide you as you try the following exercise, in which you'll look for "legacy images" that trigger insights about what's essential to you.

Set aside some quiet time, half an hour or so, in a place where you won't be interrupted. Have writing materials nearby so you can make notes.

Now settle into your body. Close your eyes and take three slow, deep breaths. Let your mind wander into your past and lead you to times when you were most yourself and episodes that shaped you. Breathe. As you see yourself then, allow random images to pop to mind—objects, places, faces, moments. (A boy on a bike. A baby's face. A desk in an office. The view from a mountaintop. A slap. A letter. Your dough- or paint-covered hands.)

When you feel complete, and you've collected four or five images, take a few more slow, deep breaths and open your eyes.

Now, one by one, think about the images you gathered, and write down the most compelling memories those images bring up for you.

Is there a particular image that inspires you or feels particularly alive? What sensations and feelings are attached to these memories and images? What do they tell you about what you most want to experience or resolve or respond to now?

Give yourself ten minutes or so to write down what comes up— more if you like—and know that you can keep returning to these images and memories over the next days and weeks to see what they reveal.

Sometimes what comes up seems enigmatic, but these "random" recollections often have an emotional resonance that becomes the seed of a legacy project.

Finally—now or after you've let your legacy images incubate a bit—turn your mind to the most recent years of your life, and muse on the questions that follow:

- What yearnings, callings, and new directions have become apparent after age sixty?

- As you think about who you are now—the person you described to yourself in your personal manifesto—what priorities and values seem most important to you?
- What small (or large) endeavor can you give your attention to today to express those priorities and values?
- Again, give yourself ten minutes, or whatever feels appropriate to you, to make notes. When you're finished, take a few slow, deep breaths to bring the exercise to a close.

In the work we've done so far, some people have seen the outlines of their legacy projects, their "rest-of-my-life's work," as they've listened to themselves in their sacred spaces, remembered old loves, or let joy carry them toward something new. For them, the answers to these questions may solidify a vision. For others, they may point toward the *feeling* of what wants to take shape.

Reflect on your legacy images and the values they speak to in you. Then resolve to take at least one small step each day toward moving those values to the hub of your life's wheel. If you feel overwhelmed by the idea of a legacy project, think of framing it as a hobby or experiment and let yourself play, always gravitating toward joy.

In the remainder of this chapter, I'll show you how other people have done that, finding their way to legacy projects that are as much gifts to themselves as gifts to the future. What you'll see are not so much revolutionary explosions into "all new lives" as much as deliberate yet thrilling unfoldings as people let themselves expand. The feeling that surrounds their projects is, at its core, celebration: "Yay! I finally get to do this!" It's a relief.

What might give you that feeling? Blue-sky it. Let yourself dream. And then let yourself *begin* and *persist* and *fall in love* with the life you're choosing.

Larry: A Hobby Becomes a New Way of Life

For Larry, the investment banker who became fascinated with woodworking, "messing around with wood" became a legacy project when he decided to build a desk. He'd been working in the woodshop he set up in his garage, struggling to master basic skills he'd been picking up from videos. There was something about the process of creating boxes and birdhouses and simple cabinets with his own hands that kept him coming back.

"I feel more like myself when I'm doing it," he told me. "I had been consumed with making money," he said, "but in my shop, I noticed how good it feels to be working with something real, something more concrete than a spreadsheet. I read books on Michelangelo, and I was inspired by the way he sculpted, the way he could see the finished product in a block of stone. I wanted to be able to do that with wood."

Larry had always admired early American furniture, and he got the idea that he'd work toward building a Shaker-style desk, something lasting and crafted, made from his time and sweat and vision. The look and feel of that furniture, its simple beauty, worked as a legacy image for him, and the desire to make it stoked his motivation to keep learning.

He sought out teachers and began to make his way more deeply into the language and tools of the craft, letting his hands absorb the ways of wood. He fumbled and failed and kept getting better at it.

Larry can be a driven guy, but woodworking has been more about process than production for him, and that shift—an attention to feeling and detail that requires being fully awake—has seeped into the rest of his life. "I'm studying Buddhism now; did I tell you?" he said. "I saw a magazine in the supermarket and picked it up," he added with a laugh, and the next thing he knew he was learning to meditate. "I've been going easier on myself," he said. "Not being so relentless, not pushing so hard. Taking one step, then the next."

It hasn't been an instant transformation. But today, eight years and countless dovetail joints in, he spends his days working on the beautiful, lasting pieces he'd envisioned. The Shaker desk, and much more, finally came to be, all the more precious for what Larry had to learn and become to make them. The satisfactions have been many. The work he does in his shop put him back in touch with the creative impulse behind his old, abandoned dream of being an engineer or architect, sculpting the world, and it connects him to the example of his laborer father. Once, he told me, he only wanted to be better than his "uneducated" dad. Now, as a fellow craftsman, he wants to be his father's equal.

Larry's sons have come to know him as a maker of beautiful things and a generous teacher—a man who's driven by love, not greed. He's lately been mentoring students at the local community college, guiding them through the basics and sharing his tools and expertise.

Larry didn't strategize his way here, he allowed himself to follow what called to him year after year, even though it didn't make sense at first. The life he has now is the one the whisper of his soul has led him to. And he has built it a day at a time after age sixty—by beginning.

Judith: Finally Answering the Call of Art

Launching a legacy project may be as simple—and profound—as finally making time for a passion that's been rationalized away and relegated to the sidelines. That's lately been the priority for my friend Judith, who spent her working life as an English teacher and then as the founder and driving force behind a magazine for nurses. She found much satisfaction in those jobs, but like many of us, she focused on career at the expense of a core part of herself she could never quite justify putting first.

Though she's been fascinated with drawing and painting for most of her seven decades, she learned as a child that "I had to finish my work before I went out to play." Art was joyful "play" that almost never found a regular place on a schedule filled with job and family duties. Ruefully she says, "I often joked that my tombstone would say 'She Worked.'" (How I related to that!)

Yet her memory is filled with vivid scenes from the rare times she brushed up against opportunities for art-making and felt herself come alive.

"I once visited the rooftop art studio in my high school after classes ended for the day," she remembers. "The spacious room was unlike any I'd seen. Most unforgettable was the light. Tall windows lined three walls; the ceiling was transparent. The out-of-doors streamed into the room. Clouds retreating from the nearby Pacific Ocean slowly floated across the sunny sky. The place positively breathed." It was a magical space that she wasn't allowed to use because there was no room in her college-track class schedule for art—and she didn't know how to insist that magic was important too. She'd put off art till college, she told herself, but when she got there, she was closed out again. Art majors got first dibs.

Finally, in her twenties, Judith studied figure drawing. "Working with charcoal in that silent room was dreamy," she remembers. Later, she bought brushes and oils, and one of the paintings she made still hangs in her living room.

In telling her story, she skips ahead to her early fifties, when "a friend and I spent a joyful two days in the woods. In the morning light, I lost myself painting leaves. My friend's occasional guidance helped me navigate watercolors, a new medium for me."

Many of us do this, connecting widely spaced dots in our histories to show how we kept deferred loves alive. Throughout Judith's work-centric years, she says, "There always was at least a thread of connection with art. Returning home from work each evening in my thirties, I invariably played piano. Intermittently over the years I drew, painted, took photos, wrote, gardened."

But the key word for her was *intermittent*, and to our wiser selves in later life, the sense of loss that comes with deferring our dreams is palpable.

"Looking back, I wonder why I didn't find another way to art, especially since my mother occasionally would set up an easel in the living room and paint for twelve hours at a time over a period of perhaps ten days. Afterward, she put everything away until the next time she felt compelled to bring out her paints again. Did it ever occur to me to ask if I could join her?"

But at seventy, Judith is discovering what it feels like to put her art first. She retired five years ago, and recently she realized that her extended family of siblings, nieces, and nephews don't need her as they used to. "I have an awareness," she says, "that for the first time in my life, my family remains central . . . but they no longer are my main focus."

She knows this is her time, and she radiates the sense of joy and possibility that comes with finally doing what she loves. She recently spent three days at a painting workshop, and came away with the breakthrough realization that she didn't have to be born with special gifts to pursue art as she wanted to—she could learn.

"This requires devotion, commitment, courage, and the firmness to gently leave the ego in another room," she says. "Some days, my courage wavers. I find myself fiddling with activities like cleaning brushes, organizing supplies, making coffee or a late lunch, checking email, raking leaves . . . anything to postpone facing the canvas. Can I mix this shade of blue again? Can I bring myself to paint over that part I love but doesn't work? Some days it's three p.m. before I dip the brush into the color before me. Settling down at last, I am absorbed for hours."

That's the truth of legacy work—it takes courage and commitment to pursue it, especially because it inevitably tips us into the uncomfortable role of being a beginner. But persisting immerses us in the satisfaction of being what we most want to be. We can lose ourselves in the process and emerge renewed.

The Gift of Giving Our True Talents

Judith is only just beginning to think of what she creates as her legacy. "I paint for myself," she says. "Over the years, I've given nine of my paintings and one photograph to people who admired them. Of the 100 or so paintings and drawings I've made over the decades, I'm pleased with some. It would be nice if family members keep a few of my images when I'm gone. But I paint for myself, to fulfill an ancient need to express myself in this way."

It can feel selfish to enjoy and express our gifts simply to "fulfill an ancient need," but doing so brings us to a way of being, and an embrace of life, that is our gift to life itself.

Choose legacy work that compels you to give your full attention with a full heart, whether you're photographing sunsets or playing music, writing, or whispering stories into the ear of a child on your lap. This is the rapture of being alive, offering your singular gifts, and nourishing yourself and the world.

"I thought that I paint only for the personal joy of it, but I didn't consider the nature, the content of that joy and how it sometimes generates a gift for someone else," Judith told me.

But that is a truth the Wise Self knows: Our most precious legacy comes from giving the world what brings us joy.

Leaving a Legacy of Compassion

Some of the most powerful legacy projects take shape as we realize that what has wounded us most deeply in life has given us the ability to help heal those with similar wounds. We have the eyes now to see ourselves in others who struggle as we once did, and to sense needs that we are uniquely able to meet. It can be profoundly satisfying— and joy-producing—to become a benefactor or mentor to them.

Bharat's project unexpectedly beckoned when he met a cheerful young man on a trip to India. Kamal was twenty-three and working twelve hours a day, seven days a week in his uncle's electrical supply store, making $107 a month, barely enough to survive. "He's an especially bright soul, quick to laugh and smile, to be positive despite having few prospects in life," Bharat said. "He left school at fourteen and doesn't have enough education to qualify for a reasonably paying job." Kamal's personality and his plight touched Bharat, and when he learned that Kamal's father had left him when he was six months old, his heart opened. That was Bharat's story, too. He decided on the spot to do what he could to help this stranger, who reminded him of his struggling younger self. "I want to do for him what my mentors did for me, to radically improve a difficult situation, in a concrete way for someone," he says. While Bharat has spent much of his life in service to others, it hasn't always been possible for him to know if his work made a lasting difference to someone, he told me. Now, he decided, he will.

Bharat leads a simple life; he is not a wealthy man. But he decided to raise $17,000 in an online campaign to buy Kamal a taxi—a chance for a new start. Bharat had never thought of himself as adventuresome, but meeting Kamal and seeing the possibility of having a significant impact on a young man's life thrilled him and diminished his fear of making his goal public and asking others to help him meet it.

"It was a stretch for me, asking other people for money, but it was a no-brainer," Bharat told me. "If I didn't respond to him, it would be a waste of a life."

The campaign has so far raised $7,000, enough for a year's worth of car insurance and a down payment on the taxi, a small, white 2018 Suzuki, which Bharat returned to India to help Kamal buy. "After three weeks of my driving and basic car maintenance instruction, Kamal has become a fine driver with an excellent feel for the car and its care," Bharat wrote to his GoFundMe contributors. "Kamal made sure that we had the car appropriately blessed by Brahman Priests at no less than seven Hindu temples."

Joy beams from Bharat's smile in photos taken on the trip. He plans to keep raising funds to help pay off the car, and to be a father figure to Kamal. That's what he wants to be remembered for, he says. "I'll always be the American stranger who stepped into Kamal's life, seemingly out of nowhere, and helped him launch a career as a cab driver."

It's the ongoing relationship, he says, that is important to him now, and I would add that whether or not Kamal's business succeeds,

Bharat's kindness and compassion constitute a legacy, an unforgettable gift that is bound to ripple far beyond his life and Kamal's.

Passing a Torch with Grace

A different sort of mentoring calls many of us as we step beyond the pursuits that once absorbed us, and want to pass on what we've learned and created. If you've mastered a skill, built a business, put your stamp on a group, or held an active leadership role, you likely want to help ensure that your wisdom benefits those who follow. For some of us, a significant legacy project involves finding satisfying ways to pass the work we have nurtured into new hands.

The gift of a graceful transition is one of the most necessary and valuable things we can give, but it can be a fraught one. The work we invested our adult lives in has a way of triggering our egos when we try to step into a supporting role, prodding us to hold onto control, or prove our worth by demonstrating how superior we are to our successors.

I learned first-hand how difficult—and satisfying—such a project can be when I realized it was time for me to cut back my involvement with Shanti. The group had evolved over the decades, and I had not been its leader for some time, but I had held onto the role of training new groups of volunteers, believing that it was important to personally transmit what I considered to be the key ideas and approach that made the group distinct.

As I moved into my later sixties, though, the trainings began to feel more burdensome, and I let myself think about turning them over to someone else. Logistically, that would be fairly easy. But personally, it was complicated. It's easy to feel pushed aside or criticized when you step back, even when the choice is yours. I had to remind myself that reducing my role wasn't the same as being put out to pasture or moving inexorably toward the glue factory. Instead, I was feeling the call of new priorities—books I wanted to write and time I increasingly wanted to spend with friends who needed me—and I needed to make room for that.

As I worked to keep my ego in check and let my Wise Self soothe it, I did my best to listen to and appreciate what my successors had to say. I'm humbled to admit that it took a while for me to realize how much insight and wisdom could come from people who didn't have my background and years of experience. But as I relaxed into simply observing, I found myself in awe of the way they were able to simplify and transmit my core teachings. Yes, sometimes I wanted to "fill out the picture." But I learned to approach such instances not as mistakes but as course corrections that *we* were making, which led to deeper understanding for all of us.

It was a test for my ego to do this, and I made many mistakes as I worked to find a satisfying relationship with the group I had given so much of my life to. Along the way I learned a number of key lessons that you might find useful as you move into a mentor-like role in the life of an organization, a group (including your family) or a young protégé, successor, or friend. To pass a torch, I've finally learned, you have to let go. These guidelines might help:

- If you're making a transition from a leadership role, look for an opportunity to maintain a defined—but loose—connection. In my case, I decided to keep attending the six volunteer training sessions my group holds every year, but to simply give an introduction, and let others do the rest. I can imagine a future where my intro talk might be presented on tape, and I just meet occasionally with the trainers.

- Make it your mission to focus on listening.
- Know that if you transmit the essence of your approach, others can fill in the details.
- Resist the tendency to offer "wise comments" and criticisms that might undercut someone's efforts and confidence in a group. Offer feedback and suggestions in private.
- At the same time, resist the tendency to step back so far you don't share useful knowledge. Work to strike a gentle balance.
- Lead with praise. Congratulate people on their efforts and point out what impresses you most. Word suggestions kindly —as options the other person might want to consider. It took me a while to figure out how not to come off like a know-it-all—especially when I had strong opinions. I learned to use words like: "You might want to try doing that a bit differently to see how it works out." I'll suggest a concrete change and end with "If you decide to try it, please let me know how it turns out. I have a feeling it might help you do X even better." Don't forget the power of the words, "I believe in you."
- Keep monitoring your tone of voice and phrasing as you stay positive in your constructive feedback: "Your presentation was terrific. I'm sure it helped the new volunteers very much. I wonder what would happen if you emphasized X even more."
- Underline the idea that you are a colleague, not an expert/ founder/revered figure to be deferred to. Use and cultivate the idea that "we're all in it together."
- Resist other people's attempts to turn you into "our beloved leader." When someone looks to me for answers, I say, "You don't need me to figure it all out. You have more than enough

experience to figure it out yourself. If you're still struggling with the same issue later on, then let's meet and work on it together."

Above all, remember that in entrusting the work you've completed to someone who can carry it into the future, you're helping ensure not only that it will live on, but that they—and you—can grow in new directions, enriched by your gifts, freed. I find that in this "emeritus" role, I feel a greater sense of satisfaction than ever before, viewing this spiritual child of mine as it grows, matures, evolves.

Allow for Changes and Course Corrections

Legacy projects, like the rest of life, don't always go as planned. Health and other crises intervene. Our interests change. Flexibility is, of necessity, part of the grand experiment.

Ellen, a member of one of my groups, had been plotting and dreaming over her legacy project for years. She's an interior designer who has long been drawn to collage art, and holds a defining memory of a period, decades ago, when she incorporated collages into journals she made for herself and her friends.

The journals have stood as a sort of legacy image for her, and anyone who knows her has heard her talk about how she'd like to conduct quarterly workshops for women, where they could collage together images of their dreams and visions for the coming season, set intentions, and renew their creative energy. When she retired, she moved to a house with an open lower level that she visualized as a "retreat space," where she could host her workshops.

But after a burst of enthusiastic planning, she found herself veering in a different direction. Her daughter, who has two small children, became pregnant with a third, and she asked for help with childcare. Suddenly, Ellen was driving fifty miles from her home every week to spend three days with her grandchildren, and she plans to be there even more when the baby arrives.

Between the time given over to travel and her regular immersion in her daughter's life, "I despair over when I'll ever be able to organize my workshops," she said. But at the same time, she added, "How could I miss out on being with the kids—especially the new baby?"

When she asked for my thoughts about what to do, I suggested something I often mention to people who are trying to balance or integrate two priorities that don't yet fit together: *Don't juggle, choose.*

Imagine that it's five years from now and that you'd totally committed to each of the possibilities, in Ellen's case either the workshops or the grandchildren.

How does it feel to have eliminated each of the possibilities from your life while embracing the other? Which of the total commitments feels most fulfilling, most joyful?

The intent here is to see if there's one choice that is right for you, while the other might be something you want to do but doesn't have the juice or bring you the same joy. Sometimes, forcing yourself to choose brings immediate clarity.

But it may not. If, like Ellen, you can't bear the thought of eliminating either choice, then focus on finding a solution that works for you, one that integrates and balances the elements that currently don't seem to fit together. The search can be its own joyful project. Brainstorm, experiment, and remain alert to the possibility that a third option that's outside the original two might emerge as a solution. Ellen realized that there were many combinations of "babies and art" that she could concoct, but that she must have both.

As you explore "both/and" possibilities, keep asking: How joyful does this potential solution make me? It may take time to find one that provides balance, but you're likely to feel bursts of the "anticipatory joy" that comes with knowing you're getting closer to the right form for your legacy project and life. Try to "hold the tension of opposites," as the Jungians put it, and wait for a solution to emerge in dreams, reveries, and conversations with others. Trust the unconscious to offer up a possibility that feels joyful and correct when the time is right.

Ellen is playing now with an idea sparked by a friend of her daughter, who talked about how she'd like to see "Ellen's retreat" someday. Shortly after, another friend suggested that Ellen might make her daughter's home her base for a while, and use her own house as an actual retreat, a place devoted to holding her workshops, focusing on her creative work, and being alone. Ellen has been trying out the idea of moving more fully into her daughter's place and using her trips home as her "collage and retreat" time.

Recently, Ellen impulsively invited her daughter's friend (and some of her own) for a weekend day of collage and conversation— not a formal workshop, but a casual creative gathering at her new "retreat space"—and she came away rejuvenated and eager to do it again. "I had been kind of overthinking it," she said. "I had built up the idea of these retreats and rituals in my mind, but it felt so good and so easy to share the art I love over wine and snacks, and for all of us to talk about our dreams and intentions. We all want to do it again soon, and invite more people. I can't wait to make journals as well. The fact is, we don't need a 'retreat,' though I love the idea. We could retreat to someone's basement and be just fine."

Undoubtedly, Ellen's project will evolve over time. Maybe it'll look just like what she began to imagine so many years ago, and maybe it will be quite different. But her devotion to finding a way to bring it to life has actively oriented her life around both of the pursuits that fulfill her and bring her joy. That's the function of a legacy project.

You Don't Have to Go It Alone

In this season of the heart, remember that legacy projects are a gift to the future, to specific others and to yourself. Although they're extremely personal, they are communal by nature, made to be shared.

In my life-review group, I was interested to see how people's interactions with friends, partners, and each other shaped their projects. At many turns, we seemed to be reminded: You don't have to do this alone.

Carl, whose dream of opening a bookstore had dogged and defeated him for many years, found himself joyfully moving forward as he talked with two close friends.

"I was having coffee with Clark and Fred and mentioned something someone in our group said, that the word *courage* means 'from the heart,'" he told me. "That sent me into another round of talking about the bookstore and how I was determined to finally have the heart to do it. It got us thinking about what we'd all like to do when we retire. Clark called me later and said, 'Before you go and find another therapist or something, how about if the three of us start a small business together, something we could all enjoy?' He said he and Fred had been talking, and they liked the idea of opening a shop in a building he's had his eye on.

"We got together, and Fred said he wanted it to be a place that sells bagels. I said it had to be something to do with books. And Clark shouted out Bagels and Books!" Carl said with a laugh of pure joy. "It sounds like a lark, but we're all serious about it. And excited. We're open to trying out the idea in a space at the temple, but I think we can actually open our own place. Whatever happens, we've got the concept: three old guys surrounded by bagels and books. It sounds idyllic to me."

Carl felt renewed and energized by the prospect, and by what could come of working with his friends to build the community he's envisioned for so long. "What could be better?" he said. "Bagels and Books."

For Tara, the fashion consultant in our group, a door to a legacy project opened at one of our meetings when she heard herself say, "I wonder how many people I've known, who I might have helped, I missed connecting with." Someone asked her for examples, and Tara immediately mentioned her sister's two twenty-something daughters, Leigh and Laurie. She'd always enjoyed seeing them, she said, but had never taken the time to engage them in deeper conversations about their lives, even though her sister had told her they were fascinated by her life and career.

"It's amazing that you can feel close to family and friends but never take the time to really get to know them," Tara mused.

"So why not do it now," one of us said. "I'll bet they'd love to have a mentor like you."

Tara teared up. "That's a great idea," she said. "You know, my Aunt Bella was so important to me in letting me see that I could be whatever I wanted to be. I know it may not happen, but I'd love to be that for them."

Tara's been arranging lunches with "the girls," and after a few meetings she reported back that she's begun to feel unexpectedly close to them. "I can't really call myself a mentor. I feel more like a combination of godmother and counselor and Aunt Bella and Auntie

Mame. I really love them, and talking to them about their choices—kids or career or both or something completely different—is helping me think about mine. We're working it out together. I'm so grateful for them. It's like nothing else in my life to see how hopeful and confident and fragile they are, all at the same time. I wondered for so long what it would be like to have daughters, and now I think I know. What a gift."

Take the Risk of Moving toward Your Dreams

The people and projects that we hunger for are often close by, but they may be more visible and obvious to friends and outsiders than they are to us. The more you share your vision of who you want to be and the values that are important to you now, the more you'll open yourself to others' insights. It takes vulnerability to do this, a willingness to say aloud, "I'm different now," or "I wonder what I've missed," or "This is what I dream of." But in my experience, it's always been worth the risk.

Devoting ourselves to legacy projects often requires a gradual, or sometimes appreciable, letting go of fear, especially the fear of not being up to the task. Many of us worry that we're not talented enough or skilled enough or smart enough or creative enough to steer toward what matters. But often, that fear boils down to the question: "Who do you think you are anyway?"

That's not a question native to the soul. It comes to us from the outside, from parents and others with fears of their own, and sometimes from an adult self who believes only winning, only perfection is enough to make a project worthwhile. When we hear that voice, which was not originally our own, we can reject it. In the moment of fear or doubt, we can breathe deeply, quieting our minds, and focus on the voice of our own Wise Self, which says: "You are certainly enough. You're equal to the task of learning what you need to know and discovering all you can be."

As you orient yourself toward whatever legacy project calls you, large or seemingly small, trust yourself, and trust this: You were born to take the risk of committing yourself fully to the gifts you dream of giving. Risk taking one small step, and then the next and the next. Feel your heart fill up.

EXERCISE:

Legacy Letters

Whatever legacy project your explorations are leading you toward, you can give your loved ones a precious gift right now by writing a legacy letter, a statement to a family member or friend of the lessons your life has taught you and the wisdom you'd most like to impart.

You can write future letters on the occasion of a significant event in someone's life, but for now, document this remarkable moment in your own life: your passage into later life. As you write, don't hesitate to tell stories or share memories of your time with the person to whom you're writing.

A simple format might be:

Dear _____,

Today, I'm X years old, and because you're so dear to me, I want to share what my life has taught me about what really matters.

First, I want you to know how much I care about you and how much I value _____ [name/describe the traits and memories of the other person that mean the most to you.]

Thank you for _____.

What I've realized as I've moved closer to old age and the end of my life is _____ . [Describe your values, the truths that you've earned and learned.]

What's most important to me now are _____ .

I will always cherish _____ . [As you think about the preceding two statements, use all your senses—tastes, smells, touch, sight—to evoke what is and what has been precious to you in this life.]

What I'd most like to say to you now is _____

_____ .

My wish for you is_____ .

You may also want to include statements like:

What I love most about my life is _____ .

What I will miss most when I die is _____ .

Rachael Freed, who has long specialized in helping people write legacy letters, suggests those last two statements as a way to get at the details you'd like to share with another person, the specifics you savor, individual as your own fingerprint. She advises spending just fifteen minutes or so on this writing, rather than agonizing over it or making it a major production. I agree. I find that a short burst of writing can take you straight to the core of what you want to say. (You can find more of Freed's suggestions and prompts for legacy letters at http://www.life-legacies.com, which I highly recommend for its wise guidance and its examples of legacy letters from a wide variety of people.) Don't be surprised if your legacy letter sparks the desire to write a memoir or create an oral history—that happens for many people.

Writing a legacy letter now, as you move toward finding or beginning a legacy project of your own, will not only help you crystallize your thinking. It will also turn your focus outward, toward potential recipients of your legacy work. Most important, it will *begin* that work, as you give the invaluable gift of love and wisdom to someone who can carry it with them both now and when you're gone.

CHAPTER EIGHT

THE EIGHTH TASK

Learn to Express Love and Accept It

L *ove heals. Love endures.* The lessons of my lifetime might well be crystallized in those four words. Love is essential throughout life, but in our later years, it gains a new centrality as the force that sustains, transforms, and makes us whole as we move through time, change, and loss.

We've been moving steadily into the territory of the heart for some time now, learning to trust what we love and to set a true course through later life by honoring what our hearts crave. Each time we do that, each time we follow our desire to paint/spend time with dear ones/offer our talents in service of someone else/gaze at the sky, we discover the satisfaction that comes with living a full-hearted life. And the more full-heartedness we experience, the harder it becomes to talk ourselves into choosing anything less. Legacy projects call us and we answer. We increasingly find ourselves choosing what inspires and feeds us over what merely keeps us busy.

Yet we're often shy about putting love itself center stage and admitting one of our heart's deepest desires: to feel a more genuine connection with the people in our lives. To reach toward them with our hopes, hurts, and all the vulnerability that later life brings requires a kind of openness that we may not yet know how to offer or receive.

One of the traps we often fall into in our adult years is valuing our own fierce independence overall, and letting friendships languish because we're too busy with "more important things" (by which we often mean work and obligations) to make time for them. Even in our sixties and early seventies, momentum and habit may still allow us to rationalize seeing a close friend or loved one only a couple of times a year because we just can't spare an hour for a drive across town. We may let our conversations with those we do see regularly become rote—health, sports, politics, kids, weather—rarely piercing the surface to get to the feelings beneath. Sometimes we stop trying to know the people whose lives connect with ours, and we don't let them truly know us.

But as we learn to pay attention to the murmurings of our hearts, many of us realize how starved we are for the nourishment of closeness, communion. Instead of fitting love in around the edges, we long to make it central. If only we knew how to close the distance we've let open up and how to find intimacy again.

Our wisdom years are our final opportunity to learn about what it means to love, and we can make a point of cultivating love now, steering toward it intentionally, teaching heart and head to work together to expand our capacity for giving love and receiving it. Starting from a base of kindness, we can soften and open ourselves to opportunities for more compassionate and meaningful relationships with the people and creatures surrounding us, both the ones we meet in passing and the ones we share our lives with. And over time, we can develop a way of relating to others that becomes less and less self-concerned and takes the form of a kind of fundamental rooting for the well-being of all. We can give ourselves over to the natural pull of the heart and connect with an embracing, sustaining love.

Love on a Street Corner

I was on the cusp of my wisdom years when Death advised me that I had been squandering my opportunities to love. The steady drumbeat of losses that took some of my closest people left me with that "intimacy with disappearance" that the poet David Whyte talks about. I was jolted out of the assumption that I would always be able to get together "later" with family and friends and share more time with them. I'd been the busy one, the tired one, the one with "important" work to do, the one who rescheduled at the last minute and shoehorned in phone calls when I was so rushed or distracted that I could scarcely take in what the other person was saying. When I thought about my father after he died, the phrase that popped up was: "Dad, I hardly knew you." We had spent precious little time getting to know each other in anything but a superficial way, and I grieved what I'd let slip away.

But I didn't really work to change the way I loved the people around me until much later, in the slowed-down months before I braved surgery for my arthritic hip in my sixties. On my many trips to the drugstore for remedies and pain-relievers, I began to pay more attention to a woman named Earlene, who panhandled outside my Rite-Aid. Earlene may not have had money, but she was queen of that corner and mayor of the block, set up on an old wooden box to offer a word, a joke, or a smile to everyone who passed, along with a running commentary on the life of the street. She was about my age, with a booming laugh and a gap-toothed grin, and every time I came by she *saw* me, human to human, and made me smile. Her energy and good cheer were genuine, a constant, and I wondered how she did it. Clearly, she was up against it financially, but she was so happy she radiated warmth.

At first I'd simply press a bill from my wallet into her hand, exchange a few pleasantries, and take one of the newspapers she was handing out. But over time, we began to talk about our lives. I asked her once how she felt about growing older, and she told me that sometimes it felt like she was losing everything, "Car keys. Teeth. Friends. Even my firstborn—he got shot in East Oakland." Her eyes filled. "To me, getting old means you're gonna lose everything you think you need to keep on living."

Then her spirit gathered itself and she continued. "Getting old is finding stuff, too. Sitting here, I find new friends—like you." That was the first time either of us had used that word, and I realized I saw her as a friend too. We began to trade stories about our pasts, and muse together on what we were both facing now. She'd come up with oddly meaningful gifts, like a fortune she'd saved from a fortune cookie—*Youth is given, maturity is achieved*—and we'd be off talking, as UPS drivers climbed out of trucks to hand her sandwiches and passers-by greeted her by name.

One day I saw her with a large-size pill dispenser and asked her about it. She had at least twelve prescriptions to sort in her pillbox, she told me. "Since you're my friend," she said, "maybe you could go along to my doctor and ask him your doctor questions about my pills."

I promised that I would—and I did. It was no big thing for me. For years I'd shuttled my mom to medical appointments, and it was easy enough to go with Earlene and figure out what was what.

It gave me great pleasure to give something meaningful of myself to help a friend who regularly lavished me with good cheer. She'd looked out for me, and I could do that for her.

My heart opened in a new way, and that's how I think connection takes hold—we notice each other, appreciate each other, and let love flow through us, moving us to express it. There are so many *others* in the world—neighbors, strangers, animal companions, caregivers, classmates, clerks. A steady stream of opportunities to turn *you* to *we*, to live in a world of closeness, of *us*.

As I felt the pleasure of this new and unexpected friendship, I knew that I needed to change the way I related to *all* the people I cared about, and to move love to the foreground. It had been easy, somehow, to befriend a stranger, but it felt daunting to think about shifting the dynamic I'd had with old friends I'd neglected or pushed away in my "busy years." Too many of them knew me as the guy who rarely checked in. Still, I was determined to try. The obvious first step was simply getting in touch again, leaving messages, making dates, sending notes: "How are you? It's been ages. How has your life been? Let me tell you about mine."

But I wanted more than a fleeting catch-up. I promised myself that I would shift my way of being with people, even on the phone, and find ways of overtly letting them know not just that I cared about them, but that I wanted to stop skating over the surface and get closer. Knowing that I couldn't just say, "I'm back! Let's be best friends," I foundered a bit. I hadn't been good about checking in or sharing my struggles, and I felt a little awkward, out of practice in the give-and-take that creates real intimacy.

But eventually it occurred to me that what I needed was "hidden" in another compartment of my life. I realized that I could fall back on the heart-centered techniques for connecting with people that I had taught to Shanti volunteers. When they meet sick and dying people, the time for connection is brief, and the hunger for closeness is acute.

It's urgent to express our caring and humanity in palpable ways that go beyond *I'm here. That means I care.*

So we developed four simple tools for building empathy, understanding, and clear communication—four ways of reminding ourselves how we wanted to be when we were with someone who needed us. It seemed a little odd to use them in my "friend life," where I thought that connection is just supposed to flow. But they helped me build closeness, depth, and love in my later-life relationships, and I think you might find them powerful as well. It might seem strange to think of friendship and closeness in terms of skills we might learn or new ways of being with those we know well. But one of the great lessons of later life is that we can find new depth in what is most familiar and experience new dimensions of love.

Four Practices to Broaden and Deepen the Love in Your Life

1. *Pause for presence*

We often move too fast and carelessly for love. Making room for it means slowing down, letting the rattle of traffic settle before we speak, and making eye contact with the other person, being fully *present* with them. This sounds completely obvious, yet it's easy to race into talking without ever bringing ourselves fully into the moment. We take it for granted that we're there when we're actually far away, still caught up in a wrangle with a bureaucrat or lost in a worry.

In end-of-life work, we consider presence to be so important that we created a small ritual for ourselves to ensure that we would be fully there anytime we visited someone. I suggested that people stop at the threshold of the room, take a few deep breaths, and visualize the connection they wanted to make with the other person. Then they'd make eye contact, say hello, and walk to the person's bedside.

Next: Pull up a chair and take the other person's hand, looking into their eyes, smiling. So simple. Yet making this kind of intentional, physical connection changed everything. In a strong, direct way, it silently communicated: *I'm here. I see you. I care.*

Meeting someone for lunch at a restaurant, going to the theater, or getting together for coffee in the kitchen is less intense than walking into a sickroom. But you can bring yourself to these casual meetings just as fully, creating warmth and actively inviting intimacy. More than 70 percent—some say 90 percent—of what we communicate is nonverbal, and you can let your body language communicate love.

A simple ritual of pausing for presence: On meeting, breathe. Make eye contact and smile broadly, pausing to silently take the other person in before you launch into a conversation or a rushed excuse for why you're late. Slow down. You might reach out both of your hands and take the other person's hands if you know the person well and are genuinely glad to see them. Notice what you see in their face. You might pat a shoulder gently. If you're huggers, you'll hug. *Feel* the presence of the other person. Feel your own.

There. You're there together.

2. *Listen from the heart*

Listening from the heart is different from being adjacent to another person while they speak. At the core it's about not just paying attention, but being willing to be moved by what the other person communicates to you and conveying your desire to engage with the emotions that come up.

What is the other person telling you with their words, body, and being? How are you experiencing it in your own body, your own heart? What are you taking in?

You may not be used to being with your friend, or anyone, in this open, receptive way, but stay with it. Our minds naturally tend to bounce from present to past and future, and in a split second our thoughts might race ahead, riff on what we might say next, or wander off on a tangent. But we can learn to notice when our minds have left the room, and when we see we've disappeared again, we can intentionally reel ourselves in. Much of presence is simply noticing the wandering—and then coming back.

Try to listen not just with your ears but with your intuition, noticing what's said and what's not, or what's being said with a gesture or an expression. Be open to whatever comes up, open to silence. Let yourself feel it.

Your willingness to simply listen, without interrupting or advising or redirecting, can feel like a rare gift to the other person, a valuing of their stories, experiences, and very being. To someone going through difficult times, the loving presence of a compassionate witness is often deeply healing. And at a joyous moment, an excited listener can amplify the joy.

The deepest of bonds are forged between those who have learned to silence their own agendas and opinions and regularly listen to one another from the heart, sharing the closeness that comes when we invite others to open themselves to us, in all their humanity—by being there to receive them.

3. *Speak from the heart*
To speak from the heart is to speak authentically, honestly, and kindly, with the goal of bringing more intimacy, affection, and acceptance into the relationship.

Sure, you'll chat about whatever you always have, but when the goal is intimacy, it makes a tremendous difference to allow the emotional and intuitive layers into the conversation. I've learned to start with affection—"It's really good to see you"—and then ask simple, open-ended questions like: "How are things going in your world?" or "What's new? Let's catch up and share what's happening for each of us since the last time we spoke." If listening from the heart to the answers means paying attention to someone's hesitation or a downcast eye (the subtext as well as the words), speaking from the heart means bringing the messages you observe into the conversation.

For me, talking with friends used to be an exchange of ideas, facts about our lives. But in these later years it's become a chance to share what's important to us now, feelings and deeper truths, and we're learning to do that more than we used to, wading in with questions that will keep us from glancing off the surface of real connection.

Instead of letting it pass when a friend seems withdrawn, as I might have in the past, I'm likely to say: "Is there anything troubling you? It looks like there might be, but I may be wrong about that." Or: "You seem distracted. Is anything going on that you'd like to tell me about?" Then, listening from the heart, I take in the response and do my best to respond with empathy and kindness.

If you're a person with a quick mind or a hair-trigger "advice response," you may be in the habit of jumping in right away with a comment, a solution to the problem someone is describing, or a story about how the same thing happened to you. But in speaking from the heart, keep in mind that people who are thinking out loud, expressing distress or excitement or describing their fears might be better served if you hear them out instead of interrupting. Letting people finish, and *then* commenting or asking for clarity, is a way of encouraging them to communicate who they are, and conveying that you're inviting them to make themselves known to you. It may seem odd to talk about speaking from the heart in terms of listening first, but as wise folk have always emphasized, nature set the balance by giving us two ears and just one mouth.

As I began making a conscious effort to offer friends more curiosity and presence, I found that it was relatively easy to move from surface chatter to deeper conversations, and to enjoy both. I began to feel more comfortable asking questions intended to get to the heart of things—"What's going on in your life that excites you?" or "Are there any challenges that I can help with?" and I discovered that most people seemed to be craving a kind of depth and authenticity and were happy to open up and answer candidly.

Even if someone dodges such questions and doesn't answer them directly, the attempt opens the door to a new level of intimacy and makes it more legitimate to express sincere concern for each other's well-being. The more comfortable I get with deeper conversation, the more comfortable the other person seems to get. The keys for me are listening and speaking from the heart, which always pull me back to presence and compassion. When I can offer those, the other person seems to gravitate toward depth and closeness.

Speaking from the Heart as a Way of Savoring

One of the great arts, and pleasures, of speaking from the heart is learning to ask questions that draw out another person so you can share more, relish more together, be there more for one another.

In his book *Curious?: Discover the Missing Ingredient to a Fulfilling Life*, the psychologist Todd Kashdan describes how sharing important experiences with someone else highlights or "bookmarks" them in our memory, lifting them out of the endless river of events in our lives and allowing us to savor and reexperience them. The interest and excitement of a listener can enhance our enjoyment and deepen the meaning of what we've lived through, whether it happened just now or years ago.

For instance: "You really did it? You brought a puppy home from the shelter? That's great! Tell me everything! I want to hear every detail." Responding with passion and curiosity says in essence, "I can hear your excitement, and I'm excited too. I want to be in the thick of it with you!"

Contrast that with a friendly but more disinterested response like: "That's great. You've been talking about that a long time. What's its name?" You can feel the energy drain away.

Kashdan points out that though we often think that being there for people in difficult times makes them feel most cared about, but actually, it's our response to their passions and positive times that makes them feel most understood and valued.

He suggests that when we hear someone telling a story about something that excites them, we bring ourselves into the experience by:

- Listening with empathy.
- Reflecting their enthusiasm back to them as they are expressing it, and doing this in a genuine way, without faking it.
- Pushing for details: "How did it happen? How did you feel? I want to hear everything!" By asking the other person more and more detailed questions as the story unfolds, you can, as Kashdan puts it, "stretch out their interest" and let the intensity and enjoyment build for both of you. The goal is to savor, feel, to be there with them, sharing their joy and excitement.

- Mentioning the story later, unprompted. Doing that shows you heard them and that it's meaningful. The continued savoring will draw you closer still.

Our stories are markers of what has made us who we are, and sharing them this way lets us hold the maps to each other, the ones that help us make each other home. In later life, as our minds lead us into the past to reexamine who and what we've been, it's natural for us to replay significant moments, and perhaps find new meaning and fresh enjoyment in them. Listening to and savoring someone else's stories is a gift of great love.

4. Act from the heart

To act from the heart is to let yourself be moved to action by caring, compassion, and your intention to be of service. As we attune ourselves to other people, becoming more present to their joys and hopes, fragility and fears, we begin to notice more opportunities to show our affection and caring. We realize it's within our power to enhance their sense of well-being, and we're drawn to do it in ways large and small. It's not that we appoint ourselves superheroes to swoop in and solve other people's dilemmas, proving to them and ourselves how loving and competent we are. Acting from the heart is less dramatic (and ego-driven) than that. Its aim is closeness and *service*, not rescue, and that means putting the other person first, honoring their desires, and always making a point of orienting yourself as a loving friend and equal.

The question, "What sort of life would I lead if I let myself act from the heart?" can prompt us to seed our lives with small, everyday practices of kindness and tender care for others, even when we "haven't been that kind of person" before.

I did this by making a series of small, regular attempts to show that I wanted to be part of people's lives. Not grand gestures but ordinary expressions of caring that I'd been neglecting: calling to suggest that we get together soon (and offering a couple of starting-point dates); remembering birthdays and anniversaries; making a point of asking about what mattered to them and remembering what they told me so I could bring it up the next time we met. Checking in by phone. Sending notes and cards by regular mail.

Each time I got together with someone, and I paused for presence and remembered to listen and speak from the heart, I was letting them know that I was not the distracted, often-distant friend of old. But perhaps most significant in shifting the ground between us was being overt about my need for them, and direct about my intention to make emotional closeness and love more prominent in the relationship.

"I'd Like to Be Closer to You."

I believe that many of us feel the urge to change the terms of our relationships in our wisdom years. We may have dotted our lives with golfing buddies, book group friends, friends from yoga/work/spiritual practice, longtime members of the same social circle—people with whom we could share activities and successes even while holding ourselves apart and making a point of showing how independent we are. That made sense as long as we also clung to the pervasive adult story that independence is all, and that we could and should be able to handle whatever came up by ourselves, without leaning too heavily on others or even necessarily letting them see our pain and struggles.

But of course, independence has always been an illusion. As our life reviews and gratitude work show so clearly, even if we're the most lonesome of the lone wolves, we can't separate ourselves from the effects of forces outside us (good or ill) or from the currents of benevolence that have arisen, unbidden, to carry us. We've *always* been interdependent, joined to the people around us, needing them as they need us. In later life, we realize we can't always handle "big things" alone—the loss of a loved one, the end of our work life, illness, and the challenges of an aging body. We're all dependent on others, and this is the normal and healthy way of living a fulfilling life. It doesn't mean that we're "less than" because we need others to get through tough times. In fact, we need others during *all* times, tough and otherwise. Seeing that, it seems natural to strengthen and repair our webs of connection.

As we feel our own vulnerability, we recognize it in others, and it moves us. And when we reach out of our isolation or insecurity to offer the healing balm of love, we discover that we can bask in the warmth that is returned. In words and with our presence and actions we begin to say: "Come closer—I want to know you." "You matter very much to me." "I care deeply about you." "You can count on me when times get tough." The narrow world of I/Me/Mine widens into You/We/Us.

I had never been an "I love you" person with those in my circle, and I told myself it was something I didn't need to do. I didn't want to be that guy who's always tossing off a meaningless "love ya." But as I got more serious about wanting to elevate love in my relationships, it made sense to me to *use* the word—after all, language structures consciousness. So "love" began to pop up in my communications with family and friends.

When I asked myself, "What can I offer now, in this minute?" I realized that often what was needed was a hug and a heartfelt "I love you." A way of saying, "I'm with you in this," whether the "this" was joy or difficulty. I've noticed with a smile that even some of my most reserved male peers, old guys like me, have learned to offer a hug, write *Love* at the end of emails, and even to say "I love you" at times when the context makes it comfortable.

Saying "I love you" can be a squirm-inducing leap for some people. Yet when we free ourselves to speak our hearts, the emotional release those words can bring can feel like the breaking of a dam. We didn't say "I love you" in my family when I was growing up, and when I first told my mom that I loved her as I cared for her at the end of her life, she looked startled then pleased, as if I'd given the greatest gift possible. It's as though she hadn't given herself permission to say those words to me—but by taking the lead I'd opened the door for her.

For many of us in later life, there is a kind of "If not now, when?" feeling about expressing and trusting love. As long as we wait, it's as if something vital has been suppressed, denied, or withheld and, as time goes by, the distress over this "holding back" intensifies. The relief and joy can be powerful when we seize the chance to put our feelings in words.

Sometimes what needs to be said is, "I hold you as one of my trusted inner circle"—something I learned as I watched my wife Cindy draw her tribe closer.

"I was never confident about how to make friends or keep them," she says. "I never understood why some people wanted me as a friend and some people who I'd like to be friends with didn't seem to be interested. This dates back to junior high school."

So, after some of the losses of the wisdom years, she found herself making a list of her friends, and asking herself which of those she could "Call at three a.m. if I needed to, and who felt they could call me" if something happened and they found themselves engulfed in emergency or fear or distress. Talking with friends overtly about how she wanted to count on them, *wanted* them to be that close, and wanted to be there for them, brought all of them comfort and drew them together. Cindy is also spending more time on incidental conversations—with the mail carrier, the checkout clerk, people walking their dogs, enjoying those sorts of small human connections. We can cultivate closeness across our lives, even if we think we've lost the thread.

A Few Concrete Ways to Start

For me, making the transition from "always busy" to "I'd like to spend time with you" was liberating. All along I'd felt bad about missing chances to connect, even as I was "sure" that my work was so very important. But as I began to reach out, I realized with joy and relief that friends and family were still willing to reach back. And I was finally ready to put them first.

Especially if you're still in the working world (or tend to get caught up in busyness), ask:

- Which of my close people needs me now?
- Who might I connect with in a way that would bring joy and meaning to our lives?
- What kind of mini-connection—a phone call, a letter or card, an email—would communicate affection to someone I feel close to?
- When might I suggest getting together for a meal/ conversation to catch up?

I now put my personal "appointments" on the same calendar as my work meetings or deadlines to give them equal importance. And if I have to cancel a personal meeting, I immediately suggest alternative dates to make it clear that I'm sorry to postpone, and that the date is important to me. Saying yes to the importance of friendship means saying no to the assumption that work ALWAYS takes precedence over personal life. In our wisdom years, there is a growing sense that integrating the two makes for a happier and more meaningful life. I love the fact that my calendar has at least as many personal "events" as work related ones—and, in some weeks, more.

Some Ideas for Reaching out beyond Your Usual Circle or Habits:
"Practice" first: I was a little nervous about offering and asking for more closeness from those around me, so I used the simple trick of visualizing myself expressing my loving feelings toward the other person several times before I did; a kind of mental rehearsal. It's a way of letting the brain experience something new and become familiar with it. If you're nervous too, I recommend using your imagination to help make you more comfortable.

Send a card: With some friends, I did one more thing: I wrote a note. I'm a big fan of sending cards, particularly the beautifully designed ones that feel like presents in themselves, something the recipient will want to keep. My messages often went something like this:

> Dear . . . , I hope you get as much pleasure from receiving this card as much as feel in writing it. I really enjoy the time we spend together, and I've been thinking about how much I appreciate knowing you. I consider you a close friend, and I'd love to spend more time with you. I'm sometimes a bit anxious about sharing my feelings with you, but I'd like it if we opened up more with each other. It's a joy to know

you and I hope we can have an even deeper relationship in the future. For now, I hope you count me as a good friend. Love and Blessings,
Charlie

Consider three people in your life to whom you'd like to say, "I love you" or "I want to be closer." Write the words in a card or a note first. Then say them face-to-face or on the phone and let each person know how grateful you are that they are in your life.

Bringing Our Closest Ones Closer

Love evolves, even with longtime partners. It can feel like a significant shift to bring heart-centered ways of communicating into relationships that may have slipped into comfortable shorthand assumptions and routines. To pause our habitual ways of being and begin to listen and speak from the heart may feel disruptive, even risky, when it moves us toward new ways of being with each other. But it opens us to the possibility of ever deeper connection when we're brave enough to acknowledge that that's what we desire.

Being with each other from the heart can be sanity-saving as later life hurls challenges our way. Partners go from seeing each other "after work" to being together much of the time. Downsizing brings people into closer proximity, redistributing the territory. Interests change. One partner may "become much more spiritual" while another may not move into spirituality at all. There's a need to negotiate roles as caregiver and patient when one person becomes ill. All of these shifts and twists can put strains on longtime love that can be fundamentally eased with an openness to listening for the emotions coloring the situation and responding to them with words and actions that come from the heart.

For my friend Jim, who recently retired at sixty-seven after a long and successful business career, the changes have come thick and fast. While his wife Jane, who is ten years younger, stays busy in her psychotherapy practice, Jim has taken a larger role in shepherding the couple's two adopted teenage kids. He's not just Dad; he's chauffeur, house manager, and internet monitor. Jane has happily turned those responsibilities over to him, but Jim is stressed, and they asked if I could help them ease the tension that's been building between them.

As I listened to them each describe what was going on, I heard Jim struggling with this change in identity. Without his profession, he felt aimless and robbed of purpose. What was he doing, just taking the boys to soccer practice and waiting to take them home? he asked. And Jane, who had long juggled care of the kids with her practice, still smarted with old resentments about the child-rearing burdens she'd carried. She wouldn't have traded her time with the kids for anything, she said, but now that Jim was retired, it was only fair that Jim be parent-in-chief until the boys were off to college. She had earned a break.

Underlying everything was their concern about how they were weathering the transition as a couple. I suggested that each of them refuel and ground themselves in the forgiveness and gratitude work that you read earlier in this book. That's some of the most useful work we can do on our own to clarify feelings and begin to address and mend longstanding issues that can run through a longtime relationship—the words "thank you," "I'm sorry," and "I forgive you" can go a long way toward helping us move forward with wholeness restored.

I urged Jane and Jim to focus as a couple on the healing and context-shifting practice of expressing love. Each person had much to appreciate about the other, and even on the busiest of days, there was time to pause to put love on the agenda. As a starting point, I suggested that they ask each other the following questions, listening from the heart to the answers, and giving a heartfelt response:

- How can I best care for you in our current situation? What do you need from me?
- How can we deepen our love for each other as our lives and family shift during these transitional years?

As well, I asked them to take turns in offering the other a unique expression of love as they each answered the questions:

- What do I appreciate about you?
- What are the ways I love you even more now than when we met?
- What do I cherish about you now that I didn't see in our earlier life together?
- What are my hopes for our future together?
- How does your love sustain me as we grow older together?

It's easy for a loving couple to lose sight of one another in times of change. Pausing to express love and the practice of being together from the heart can reset a connection, especially when people are committed to learning and speaking the language of loving care. I'm an ardent advocate of counseling when tensions are severe, but I have often seen the power of simple, constant acts of love to close the distance that's opened up between people.

Jim and Jane found, as they talked, that they were both in the midst of finding the right balance between self and family, work and mission, but that feeling the other's appreciation and support for their contributions energized both of them. And when they drew their kids into the discussion for a family circle, Jim was especially heartened to hear how much his boys loved having him there. Even when they seemed to chafe or to tune him out, he realized, "It's a big deal to have their old man around."

The remarkable thing about love is that we can ask for it, *talk* about it, and bring it to the foreground, rather than expecting that it will take care of itself. We can feed it. Nurture it. See it thrive.

Radical Love

I feel blessed to have what I consider to be a soul-mate relationship with Cindy. My most ardent and frequent expressions of love go to her, and it's as if I want her day to be as good as possible and by expressing my love I believe I can make that happen. One of the images I cherish is of the two of us holding hands when we walk and at times at home as a way of expressing a kind of loving Oneness. She's always saying that we're a unit, like two trees connected at the root but with different appearances above ground.

I say this simply to suggest that this variety of love too is possible, and that we can choose to make ourselves part of a loving unit with friends if we don't have a partner. We can call each other family and weave ourselves into each other's lives, eating together, traveling together, being there for each other with kindness and regular expressions of love.

Lately I've been thinking about what I call "radical love." The word "radical" comes from the Latin word *radix*, which translates as "from the root," and I think of radical love as one of the sweetest manifestations of love in our wisdom years. As life slows down with age for longtime friends and partners, we see who they really are, what they value, what they are at the core. Radical love is a sense of gratitude and appreciation for a person simply for being. It's natural to feel a love that flows from all another person has done for you, all the care and acceptance and love they have given. But radical love, as I experience it, is a glow of joy that says, "I'm so grateful for who you are, that you ever came to exist in the first place, and that we've found each other in this life."

This is love at its most expansive and most accepting, and it's one of the finest gifts we can offer another person—and ourselves. It becomes possible when we truly get that the quality of our life is enhanced by the presence of the other person. And it blooms when we let them know how precious they are.

The catch to this kind of love is that it can only be as deep as the love we offer ourselves. Only when you love yourself as a decent, caring, and compassionate human can you see and appreciate those qualities in someone else. All of the work you have done until now, all the forgiveness and gratitude you've offered others and yourself, all the joy you have allowed yourself to experience, all the excitement you've found in your own passions and your deeper self, have brought you to this place of being truly able to love.

Taking Love into the World

Love is an expansive and self-replenishing force that can restore us even in the midst of a time when loss finds us more frequently than before, and our circle of close ones begins to scatter and contract. Comfortable and comforting opportunities to share love may seem to shrink as kids move away, friends and relatives die or are lost in a jungle of health concerns, and our own mobility diminishes. We can find ourselves left with more time at home, perhaps alone. But such changes give us time to reflect. And we see more clearly than before that love is the treasured essence of what has mattered to us, and what matters now.

Who have you loved most? Who has loved you? Love is the gift we remember above all as we look back on our lives, and it's the most precious thing we have to offer in the time that remains to us. What would happen if you moved it to the center of your life now, seeking every opportunity to express it? Who would you call? What small kindness would you offer from the heart? What caring chance would you take with the next person you meet? How might you become an artisan of love, honing your skill at expressing your love to more and more people and animal companions?

When love becomes a priority, our days and choices begin to revolve around our sense of how love can connect us with everything we see, and we begin to perceive the world and the beings in it as potential recipients of our love. Simply moving through the world in a heart-centered way—listening, speaking, and acting from the heart—can place us in a flow of love that fills us up with the satisfaction of giving and receiving. We become increasingly sensitive to who needs our love and how best we might express it to them, both those who we count as dear and those who suddenly come into view once we slow down enough to notice them.

Judith, who is savoring her talents as an artist in her wisdom years, told me about a trip she and a friend took recently to Point Reyes Station, a small tourist town in northern California. A man sitting on a low wall in front of the post office looked up as they went by and said, "Can I show you my art?" They paused and the man began flipping the pages of a small, worn sketchpad, its edges turned up, smudges on some pages.

The quality of the work surprised her. "There were colored pencil drawings of mythical figures, landscapes filled with imaginary beings, each one exquisitely detailed with an amazing use of color," she remembers. "'These drawings are beautiful,' I told him. 'You have so much talent.' He lit up and began to turn the pages faster to show us more, pointing out details on each page. We stood there, admiring and talking about the work for at least ten minutes." Judith was curious about the work, engaging him artist to artist, and as she and her friend walked away, Judith told her friend, "His sketch pad is nearly full. Let's get him a new one."

They stopped in every gift shop in town, as well as the bookstore and hardware shop, looking for a pad or book with blank, unlined, textured paper, and when nothing just right turned up, they returned to one of the gift shops, this time asking a clerk if she had a small journal. "Just one, on a bottom shelf at the back of the store," the woman said. It was the perfect sketchpad, bound in thick leather embossed with a mountain.

They had it wrapped and took it back to the man at the wall, who nodded at them and tossed the parcel onto the backpack and bedroll beside him. Judith encouraged him to open it, and as he did, his eyes filled with tears to see a gift that was clearly chosen for him, something that honored his work and encouraged more. He knew he'd been seen as the artist he was. "Before we walked away, he wrote down for us his name, his nicknames, and his mother's contact information. He told us his name was Billy, that he had inherited a farm in New Hampshire, and was moving there soon."

Judith has always been a giving person, but the nature of the contacts she makes is different for her now, she says. "Knowing myself better and understanding more of what it is for people to live this life, I see others more deeply as human beings in the full array of emotion and circumstance." As for so many of us in later life, it's become easier for her to see the human in front of her, to ask, "Who is this person?" and to make a loving connection, instead of one that is dutiful or superficial.

"These encounters can be gift-giving fests," she says. "Billy gave us the gift of being open with us in sharing his work, inspiring us. We in turn gave him the gift of seeing him and interacting with him beyond his homeless situation, of engaging with him as the artist he is."

As we experience the world through the heart, it becomes a more intimate place filled not with distance and strangers but with love and moments of genuine connection.

Love and Grace in Difficult Times

I've been amazed and inspired over many years to see the way love can expand a life even in situations where a person's world seems to have been reduced to the space around a sickbed. There, I've seen how love, expressed in the moment and savored in memories of the past, is larger than pain, larger than fear, large enough to absorb and transcend them. The richest of us are those who freely give away the best of who we are—our loving selves, our caring, our appreciation for others.

Love—and its close companions, gratitude and forgiveness—brings grace to the hardest times. "I'm sick, yes, but what a delicious breath. Look at the sky. I savor this memory, this moment, this person's touch. The magnificent stars still shine over my bed and the night sky after the funeral is a miracle. My heart aches and oh, the light in that tree, the purr of the cat, this music, this love I carry inside."

We can't always cure the partner's memory loss or the money troubles or the loss of mobility. We can't reverse time and its effects. But we can cultivate joy in the midst of it, love in the midst of it. We relish our good times and deal with the tough ones with the power of the heart and spirit. We can reach to our depths, reach toward others, and replenish ourselves with love.

CHAPTER NINE

THE NINTH TASK

Open to the Eternal

As we tend to the tasks of transformation that draw us closer to our Wise Selves, we begin to wake up to the worlds inside us. Both outwardly and inwardly, we are becoming less tethered to the habitual demands of jobs and families and the busyness of old routines. And as our bodies and the pace of our lives slow, many of us feel drawn to solitude and reflection, returning to our center, touching the ground of the soul. Standing in the still, holy place at our core, we begin to commune with the expansiveness of love and beauty and the aliveness of our purpose—as well as whatever else we think of as God.

Longing for wholeness, I believe, we all become spiritual seekers in later life.

When we sit with Death at our shoulder, we begin to realize that we're ancestors in training, leading the way for the young who follow. This is the opposite of what's usually posited, that the young are carrying us into the future and are the bearers and builders of what's important. That line of thinking, which is so much a part of our mindset as ambitious adults, misses seeing what becomes so apparent in our later years: What make us fully human are our highest values—resilience, peace, and fulfillment, as well as gratitude, forgiveness, compassion, and love. *This* is the ancestral wisdom we transmit by example to those who come next. And to embody that wisdom, we must enter the realm of the spirit, the soul. That draws us into an ever-closer relationship with the eternal.

We sometimes think of our dance with the eternal in terms of the imprint we will leave on those we've touched, who will touch others in a chain whose end we cannot see or imagine. But I believe that we also find ourselves in a relationship with the Mystery that is far greater than our ego selves or our bodies. We've had glimpses of it all along, when we've fallen deeply in love, or felt profoundly moved by another person, a work of art, a piece of music, a contact with nature—times when we seem to dissolve into something that transcends us. These are experiences that we've been cultivating in our journey so far, experiences that tell us there is more to us, more to life, than meets the eye. This "more" is our timeless being.

Harriet, the psychotherapist, found herself in unexpected conversation with the Mystery after cutting back her work hours at seventy to work on the book that she hopes will capture all she's learned in her long career. When writing didn't feel alive and joyful to her, she began spending increasing amounts of time outside in the garden she'd always left to someone else's care. It was a compelling diversion to have her hands in the dirt and watch plants go from seed to sprout to flower to bare stalk. But gradually, the time she spent tending and watching and weeding became central to her, a window that illuminated both the outer world and the one deep inside. "Nature's beauty is inspiring, and I want to help it along," she told me the other day. "Sometimes I'll look at a flower and feel like I'm looking at God's face." She knows I know she's never been religious or talked about God, and she laughed to see my surprise. "It's funny," she said, "how there's so much more to life than people's problems."

Returning to the Questions

It can be startling to notice our minds drifting toward the Mystery and searching for meaning there if we haven't been much concerned with spirituality, or if it's been many years since we examined what we believe. But I've noticed that the veil between us and the eternal begins to thin as we grow older, and we become curious about the deeper dimensions of our lives. We feel drawn to understand both the eternal—the realm of life that unfolds outside of time—and eternity, which we often imagine stretching into a future without end, a dimension in which we might experience an afterlife, heaven, reincarnation, reunion with loved ones, or some other reality.

Whatever we thought we'd concluded earlier in life, questions about what we believe gain urgency as we watch loved ones suffer and die, and we face the reality of our own losses and death. Some of us have absorbed the beliefs of childhood religions, whether we still practice or not, and understand questions of the Mystery through the stories of the traditions we grew up with.

We've felt our way into or away from spiritual life, influenced by our cultural traditions or college philosophy classes or late-night bull sessions or mystic teachings or drug experiences or twelve-step work. And we've evolved with age. Our minds, hearts, and bodies know life differently than they did when we were young, especially now that we've come closer to death and seen what's sustained our loved ones through their last breaths. Now, our task is to build a relationship with the eternal that will sustain *us* through all that will come.

The Wise Self and Death ask us to sit with fundamental questions about our spirits and to put sincere effort into answering them for ourselves, letting them lead us wherever they will:

- How do you understand God and the eternal?
- Are there times when you feel closer to the divine/the eternal? What are they like for you?
- Have you had "transcendent" experiences of some sort? What can you put into words about them? Did they change the way you live?
- When you die, do you believe a part of you will live on?
- What's shaped your understanding or beliefs? Are they evolving as you grow older?
- Has your proximity to someone dying changed your beliefs?

This territory is both vast and deeply personal, and I can't begin to map it for you. But I can share a sampling of the paths taken by others, including me, and some of the questions and conclusions I've come to in my work with the dying. Perhaps all many of us can do is to live our questions about the eternal and devote ourselves to the practices that put us in contact with our deepest truths. We can keep asking, keep listening, keep living our way through the questions and feel our way toward understanding.

The Eternal: It's Not What You Think, It's What You Are

I've been chasing the Mystery ever since I was a young man. The only book I ever stayed up all night to read was called *Cosmic Consciousness*, in which a nineteenth-century British psychiatrist named Richard Bucke recounted a mystical experience that shaped his life. He'd spent the evening with friends reading poetry, and on returning home was quietly reflecting when he suddenly "found himself wrapped . . . by a flame-colored cloud." At first he thought he was witnessing a fire in the city outside, but he realized in a flash that the light was coming from *inside* him. As he puts it (writing in the third person), "Upon his heart fell one drop of Brahmic Bliss, leaving thenceforward for always an aftertaste of heaven." He suddenly knew that the universe was alive, that the soul is immortal, and that love is absolute and certain. The mystical didn't intrude on him again, but that one episode shaped the rest of his life.

Bucke got his taste of heaven at the end of the 1800s, and when I encountered it in the 1960s, it was as vivid as any episode from *The Electric Kool-Aid Acid Test*. It piqued my curiosity and my desire for that kind of intense contact with glowing cosmic consciousness. Perhaps like you, I was hungry then for a flash of illumination that would change me forever. It wasn't that I hadn't touched the Mystery. I have felt the moon as a mystical companion since I was a lonely young boy and had glimpses of the aliveness of the cosmos that let me understand Bucke's description. The experience of being immersed in the immense beauty of the Grand Canyon and amid the glaciers in Alaska; feeling a profound sense of oneness and love on a handful of drug trips with psilocybin; losing myself in the sacred space of Notre Dame Cathedral, bathed in the radiance of the magnificent stained-glass windows—each of those indelible encounters touched my core and connected me to something much larger than my body or ego.

But I longed for a *lasting* communion with the eternal. My moments of transcendence seemed like blessings, but they left me feeling like an outsider when I returned to daily life, unable to hold onto their gifts. Inside my routines, my ordinary days, the eternal seemed far away, perhaps because on some level I was hoping for some kind of perpetual ecstasy, with fireworks always exploding, symphonies ever reaching a crescendo, angels holding trumpets. I was focused on an exalted state that needed perfect conditions to emerge, a state of unending bliss.

In my wisdom years, I've looked back at my younger self's hunger for all that with a gentle smile, seeing how it suited him and his belief that *anything* could be willed into being with enough reading and thinking and planning, even the ineffable. I feel blessed by the times when I've known with visceral certainty that I am not separate from God or nature or any aspect of life, times when I've felt a unity with existence vibrating in my being. I smile at how much I wanted to cling to those moments, hold them in a freeze frame. But in these years after sixty, I've been able to hear the wisdom teachings of many traditions, which point us toward letting go. The eternal, they tell us, is here *right* now, even as we smell rain coming and close the windows, stroke the cat, see the brilliant light in the clouds. We touch it simply by being alive and awake in a moment that will never reappear and which cannot be held. I had been reaching out toward a distant eternity, not quite realizing that the eternal was something I'd find here, inside.

Eternity and the Eternal Now

One of my favorite guides through the Mystery is Joseph Campbell, who devoted his life to studying the diverse cultural stories and beliefs that capture who we are as humans, and that show how we make meaning of our lives, our deaths, and our place in the cosmos. In an unforgettable series of conversations with journalist Bill Moyers in the late 1980s, filmed for PBS and titled *The Power of Myth*, Campbell traced these stories and themes across continents and through millennia.

Whatever names and faces we give to God, he said, all of them are "the masks of eternity." Our stories, our words, will never be adequate to capture the reality of the eternal—we'll always be speaking in metaphors, hoping to describe the spiritual potential we have within us and our manifest experience of that life that pours into the world from an inexhaustible source, animating us and everything else. Our world of things and time, ego and the body, change and loss, sits atop a world of radiance that exists *beyond* time.

"The central point of the world is where stillness and movement are together," Campbell said at one point, analyzing a story from the Sioux tradition. "Movement is time, but stillness is eternity."

These are the hallmarks of the eternal, as Campbell describes it: *It is still. Beyond time. Radiant. Our true, enduring life.*

How do we open ourselves to that?

There's something key in the idea of stillness, by which I mean the stillness of the mind, a quieting of thoughts and emotions and fears and opinions about what's going on. That lets us settle into presence, or as Deepak Chopra puts it, "pure, undisturbed awareness."

"The active mind isn't the same as the still, quiet mind," he says. Putting ourselves in contact with the "field of pure awareness" puts us in contact with experience that's not bound by time.

Religious practices and ritual, prayer and meditation can give us practice in finding this stillness, this presence. There are many traditions that work with quieting the mind and releasing ourselves into the deep well of the eternal, and I highly recommend listening to wise and compassionate teachers inside and outside your own tradition to discover what practices might resonate with you now. (I'll recommend some sources I like in the reading list, and I encourage you to explore.) But you may have noticed that throughout this book we've been approaching the eternal in a variety of ways already, coming at it from many angles that may form elements of a new "practice" for you: Making space in your life for listening to the voice of your being. Gravitating toward what immerses you in joy or awe. Learning to be with people "from the heart," and cultivating the endless gratitude and generosity that flow from a place of presence and compassion. All of this can bring us into contact with the eternal that sounds through the Eternal Now.

When I ask people how they experience God/the eternal/the divine, however they define those, the specifics vary, but it's stillness, rather than fireworks, that rings.

Scenes from the Eternal: Holding a Sleeping Child

A friend of mine, Kaushik Roy, who's in his early forties, described a particular kind of divine communion that I hear many parents and grandparents speak of: the transcendent connection with a child. Kaushik, a wise old soul in a youthful body, told me how he loves to hold his four-year-old daughter, Neela, when he returns home from work. Tired, but so eager to see her, he sits back and lets her climb into his lap, holding her against his chest. "I realized soon how special and peaceful those moments are, when I hold her, rock her, and she drifts off to sleep. Those moments are as close as I have ever gotten to God."

Kaushik was brought up in a Hindu faith. He says, "I learned early in life that there is a notion of a real self that is profoundly happy; a perfect self. When I hold Neela, I am close to being desireless in those perfect moments. I need nothing else. I've never felt anything else in my life like those experiences. It occurred to me that Neela and I are in a lineage of fathers and daughters that go back into prehistory, many of whom experienced this timeless, unconditional love. I am in awe of how special and peaceful these moments are. Neela's middle name is Shanti—inner peace—and that's what I feel when I hold her on my chest at night and she dozes off. There's nothing else I need in my life than this perfect feeling, this contentment."

Question for reflection: When in your life have you experienced a perfect moment of inner peace and contentment?

Scenes from the Eternal: Disappearing into Art

Judith, who in her wisdom years is finally expressing her lifelong passion for art, describes a different path to everyday transcendence: losing herself in her painting, something she thinks of as "disappearing."

"What's always drawn me to the arts is the allure of disappearing," she says. "Disappearing never occurs to me while I prepare to paint. I never seek to disappear. It's neither a conscious nor an unconscious goal. Time in that dreamy place is total Being, without words, without separation. It's only in retrospect, after the brush is put down, that I realize where I've been."

This kind of immersion also brings us to the eternal, an embrace of our life and gifts that is our gift to life itself. Judith tells me she's been thinking about this a lot, this relationship between the personal joy of creating and the effect of that joyful pursuit on the world beyond herself.

"A couple of years ago, my spiritual teacher and I were talking when he noticed an Ensō, on a brochure laying on the table before us," she says. An Ensō is a circle painted in ink on paper with a single brushstroke. In Zen Buddhist practice, it symbolizes many things, including the moment when body and being join in a fluid act of creation.

Judith's teacher stood admiring the Ensō, and when he mentioned that he'd someday like to have one, Judith was overtaken by the desire to create one for him as a surprise (which it would be—he didn't know she was a painter). She prepared her paper and ink, and let her brush swoop through twenty-six Ensōs before the one she ultimately gave him flowed in just the right way. The evening she offered her gift, she remembers, he carried it around the meditation room, and showed it to each person on the cushions. "'This came to me at a time I needed it,' he said. And I was struck with the thought, 'This is why I was born.'"

Disappearing into her art— enveloping herself in an awareness of what's before and within her—only happens when she's fully present, standing in the eternal. "It involves painting what's inside me when in the presence of what's being painted—in other words, a reflection of what I'm perceiving and experiencing. It's a coming-together with the subject," she says, "And that is one of my ways of listening with an open heart to what's around and within me. Perhaps painting gives me an opportunity to better offer my listening to others. This is the best of myself."

Question for reflection: When have you been fully immersed in an activity that left you feeling that you'd "disappeared" into what you were doing?

Scenes from the Eternal: Waking to Magic and Mystery

The descent—or is it ascent?— into being deeply here, right now, sometimes saturates the ordinary with magic, or has a mystical feel. I've been interested to hear even the most "rational" of my friends speak in those terms. My friend John, a psychologist in his sixties who doesn't practice a religion, said he was reluctant to answer specific questions about god and divinity, but then went on to muse eloquently about them. "For me the divine opens up when I'm communing with the mystery and beauty of life—when I have an increased sense of the magical dimension of being," he told me. That connection to a larger presence happens "when I'm in nature, which includes traveling to interesting places. I was recently in Machu Picchu and the Galapagos Islands and felt a deep sense of awe and beauty. It felt humbling, inspiring, and uplifting to be in the presence of such incredible beauty and mystery.

"I also feel this connection when I am in the presence of people who are open and have the capacity to connect in a deep way," he told me. "When both our minds are relatively quiet and still, I allow myself to relish a sense of connectedness and aliveness that transports us beyond ourselves, even if for just a few precious moments."

Though some of us prefer to keep our experiences of the eternal to ourselves, it's illuminating to open up this aspect of our lives with other people, even when, as John puts it, "no clear answers emerge."

I get a sense that more of us than we know have witnessed "the magical dimension of being," as the eternal pushes through to the surface of our experience. My friend Lynn, who describes herself as spiritual but not religious, told me about having "moments of great, unexpected presence, when I felt I could truly see the world," which tapped open the door to the eternal for her.

"My college boyfriend and I used to take long, silent rides in the mountains and foothills in his old, white pickup truck," she said. "Silent is the wrong word—the motor had a low roar and the truck clanked over the rough roads, but the two of us were silent for long stretches as we looked out at the land. It's beautiful in the Rockies. Sometimes my mind would simply stop narrating, and I remember passing a stand of trees and just *seeing* them, without the idea of 'tree.' I could see and feel the light coming from them and me. We were the same glowing thing. I delight in language, but experiencing the trees that directly gave me an understanding of what words take away. It was a revelation, seeing how much bigger the world is than I thought. It's not me/it. It's *us*."

Lynn emailed me later to add a postscript to her story.

"I nearly laughed out loud when I read an essay in Annie Dillard's book *Pilgrim at Tinker Creek*, which describes almost exactly how those trees had appeared to me. Sitting on a log bridge at the creek as the sun is setting, she senses her vision shifting, and the world is suddenly radiant. She says that what she saw around her was 'like stars being born at random down a rolling scroll of time. Something broke and something opened.' That was it! I had had that same sense of something breaking open and putting me in the presence of the whole cosmos when I experienced those trees.

"I'm sure you can't will this kind of seeing, you can only wake up to it," Lynn wrote. "And waking up, Dillard says (in a much more beautiful way), seems to depend on getting the mind quiet, so its chatter doesn't stand between us and what is actually here.

"At the end of the essay (it's called 'Seeing'), she describes one other example of this way of seeing. As she's walking in the woods, her mind stops talking, and she comes upon a cedar tree, which she sees suddenly as blazing with life—'each cell buzzing with flame,' is how she puts it. She simply beholds all of that. Gradually, the tree becomes just a tree, but once she's seen it lit up with life, it changes her, the way my long-ago vision of the trees changed me. 'I had been my whole life a bell, and never knew it until at that moment I was lifted and struck,' Annie Dillard writes. Yes, I thought. That's exactly it!

"When you ask me about the eternal, that's what I think of. That's what I know I am and we are and trees are. We are, right now, blazing with life. And sometimes we can see it."

Question for reflection: When have you had an experience of waking up, when the eternal pushed through to the surface of your everyday experience?

From the Eternal to Eternity and the Afterlife

So all of this blazing, immersive, awe-producing, love-filled *life* we connect to when we still our minds and find ourselves in this eternal now, all this energy that comes to us and through us, connecting us with all that is—what happens to it when we die?

I have walked through the dying time with strangers, and with those I love the most, and found that all of us, as our time grows short, reach toward our own understanding of what happens to the spark that will be gone from our bodies when our hearts stop beating. And no matter what we thought before, as we near the last chapters of our lives, we want to come to terms with the vastness we confront as we look at and beyond death. Is it empty? Full? Is it empty of *us*? We need to answer for ourselves: What comes next?

It's easy to table thoughts about the afterlife when we're younger, but Death, that adviser who's been prodding us to take the risk of coming alive in the time we have left, now turns our focus to the fast-approaching horizon, pushing us to ask again: Is this life all there is? Is there an afterlife? Will some part of me live on? What do I really believe?

These questions become more than just cocktail party chatter or workshop deliberations, with death's reminders coming closer. In part, we need to find answers for ourselves to ease our anxiety about dying. But I think we also realize we can't navigate these waters with only a child's conception of heaven or a young adult's cool and removed perspective. By now we've lost parents and friends, faced our own mortality and fragility in numerous ways, and we bring not just received wisdom to our inquiry about death, but also memory and proximity and sometimes even the experience of dying, or coming very close, ourselves.

The possibility that there might be more in store for us beyond this life presents itself urgently and compellingly to many of us at the very end, regardless of what we thought before. Even my best friend Rico, an intellectual rationalist with no interest in spirituality, said, just before he died: "I think we'll meet again." I've heard final words like that from people much like Rico again and again.

We have time now to consider our beliefs, our hopes, and all life has taught us about the eternal. Between the certainty of those who say, "I know there's nothing more than this," and the ones who will tell you, "I know what corner the afterlife is on, what color it's painted, and how late it's open," comes a whole lot of questioning. And we questioners are enriched by the asking.

A 2018 study by the Pew Research Center reported that 50 percent of the Americans it polled said they were somewhat or very religious, and 71 percent called themselves somewhat or very spiritual. Eighty-nine percent said they believe in God (56 percent said they believed in the God of the Bible while 23 percent believed in another "higher power"). I was fascinated to see that 71 percent of the respondents, whether "religious" or "spiritual," believe in heaven and 60 percent believe in hell. A third of them believe in reincarnation. And I wondered what these many people envision when they use words like *heaven* and *reincarnation* and *hell.*

When Joseph Campbell talks about the afterlife, reincarnation, or resurrection, he makes a point of saying that the stories of our religions—our myths—are to be interpreted symbolically. Heaven?

A symbol. Reincarnation? A symbolic image. Symbols of what? The depth of the eternal that we can experience right here, right now, by reaching within for renewal and bliss and resurrection and rapture. We can make contact with the mystery that we are, Campbell might say, and let it come through us, casting off limiting personalities, bringing our fullness to light, pouring life into life.

When you say reincarnation or heaven or afterlife, what do you visualize? What do you really mean? When was the last time you put words to what you believe?

Our Own Wisdom: Everyday Perspectives on Death and the Afterlife

I've been deeply moved, excited, and illuminated by hearing about the experiences that have led other people to their beliefs and shaped their ideas about death and what might lie beyond. Though many of us avoid talking about religion in our day-to-day conversations, this protective reflex can cut us off from precious insights into one another and keep us from passing on some of the most profound learnings of our lives. I'm convinced that sharing our questions, and feeling our way together toward answers that often seem more like *openness* to truths rather than a *grasping* after them, is the way to peace and wisdom.

To that end I'd like to offer a few of the responses I got when I asked a small collection of people to share their beliefs about what, if anything, lies beyond this life. These voices have resonated in my mind and heart and fed my own questions and answers. I hope they will do the same for you.

Scenes from Death and the Afterlife:
John—Open to the Mystery

My friend John, the psychologist, had no ready answers about the afterlife, and he was comfortable with that. He's nondoctrinaire in life, and that's the approach he takes to death. "For me, what we call 'God' is both transcendent and immanent," he said, "an intelligence, or presence, or reality that lives beyond our usual sense of self, yet can be experienced in a bodily felt way if we can get quiet enough to notice it, allow it, relish it, and let it swirl through us for as long as it wants to last. It's an experience of grace that we cannot control, yet we can create an inner environment where it is more likely to arise."

Does that experience of grace disappear when we die, or does it go on and on? John didn't speculate. "For me, the key is to just be open for the adventure and journey. To just remain curious and not cling to any certainty about an afterlife or what it might be like. I'm hoping there is a vibrant and connected afterlife for me and others, but I'm not sure about it . . . or anything in that realm. I just try to stay open to possibilities and to embrace the mystery of it all."

Question for reflection: What, if any, is your conception of the afterlife?

Scenes from Death and the Afterlife:
Micaela—Dying and Coming Back

Micaela, who's in her early sixties, is the director of a crisis hotline in New York and is never far from the crossroads where death and life intersect. "I train people to sit with people who are questioning life and their existence," she said. "I talk to people almost every day who are wondering about what happens after this life. They wonder about loved ones they have lost to suicide, traumatic death and 'natural' deaths. I also talk to people who are facing the end of their lives. I am just open to the discussion. I am able to listen to people talk about what is frightening. That is a gift I have had all my life."

Her perspective on death, and her ability to listen compassionately, have been informed not only by this work, but also by her nearness to the deaths of others and her own near-death experience. Three years ago, while undergoing surgery for a septic gallbladder, she was pronounced clinically dead. She said that in the moments after her body systems stopped, "I experienced abject joy and the realization that I could 'just go.' I experienced myself expanding into a field, my molecules dissolving and diffusing.

"I was given a choice to stay or go," she told me. "I received the information that if I left, my partner would have a much harder time coping with what was coming for her. Reluctantly, I chose to stay for her, knowing that when I do leave this mortal coil, it will be joyous."

Micaela doesn't dwell on the details of what an afterlife would look like. "The Law of Conservation of Energy states that energy cannot be created or destroyed in an isolated system. I believe that," she said. "My body will die and my consciousness will continue in some way in other realms. I am suspicious of the 'white light' [that some people report seeing in near-death experiences]. I wonder if it's a trick to recycle us back into this three-dimensional matrix. I really don't care about seeing dead relatives or anyone else for that matter." She keeps her focus on being of service, living in conscious and ongoing communion with the divine.

"I feel closer to the Beloved when I stop what I am doing. I deliberately go slower, and pay attention. If I am driving, I sing to the Beloved," she said. "If I am waiting in line or in a meeting or watching a movie, I pay attention to my breath and say silent *japa* on my prayer beads (repetition of the many names of the Beloved.) Then I smile, at my own self. Doing this reminds me that 'everything is all right.'"

Micaela told me that while she has long been a student of Eastern teachings and philosophies, work with people at the end of their lives has deeply affected her belief system. "As I have grown older, I have let go of a lot of dogma and taken the 'let's see what happens approach.'" she said.

"After a lifetime of self-inquiry, reading the works of philosophers, sitting at the feet of many masters, being with many people at the end of their lives and having a near-death experience myself, I am serene with the idea that God, the Divine, the Source of all, is my own self. God is as close to me as my own breath," she said. "No matter what happens, everything is all right."

Question for reflection: What is *your* conception of God, the Mystery, the Ground of All Being?

Scenes from Death and the Afterlife:
Maria—Discovering What Lives On
Maria, a Buddhist spiritual teacher in her sixties, traced her understanding of what happens after death from her childhood religion to her current Zen practice. "In my youth, the Church was my guide to an afterlife with the Trinity," said Maria, who'd been sure as a devout Catholic child that she would grow up to be a nun. "In early adulthood, I leaned on the philosophical underpinnings of Enlightenment, evolution of the species to include god-like qualities around expanded consciousness (a love of the mind.)" But toward the end of her long career as a scientist and businesswoman in the medical and biotech fields, the work that had consumed her began to seem hollow, and as she left it behind, her beliefs evolved again, becoming

less rooted in the mind. "My sense of the divine became neither other person-centered, nor self-focused but grew toward a universal presence, a presence that is at heart compassionate and incorporates all being."

To explain what that means to her, she described an experience at an extended meditation retreat: "I became very concentrated, very still. At some point, while being aware of what was occurring around me, people arriving and leaving the room, talking, and so on, I recognized I was in an altered state of consciousness. There was a sense of no boundaries between my body and all the other energy in the room and beyond. As I was sitting there, watching this, I was overwhelmed by a profound sense of contentment. It felt like a divine blessing; in another context, I would have called it grace. The phenomenon lasted several hours. It was not something I held, but participated in. Afterward, as consciousness returned to normal, all I wanted was for everyone to experience this level of contentment sometime in their lives."

Yet maintaining any particular state of consciousness isn't the goal. Recently, Maria cut herself badly with a kitchen knife while cooking, and witnessed herself in the moments before she fainted. "When it happened, despite all my efforts to stay conscious, it was a light going off. I was conscious and then I was not. And then I was. In the interval during which my body kept breathing, I was not aware of my surroundings, or even the fact that I fainted. I was not there. It was a succinct reminder that I am not my consciousness," she said.

Maria has worked with the Zen Hospice Project in San Francisco and watched her own loved ones die, and all this witnessing of herself and others has contributed to the understanding of life and dying that she holds today: "At death, I don't believe I will go anywhere or become something else. My body will cease being animated: breathing, blood circulating, muscles twitching. Consciousness will cease, also," she told me. "Whatever constitutes the life force in me will still exist, but be irrelevant to the person who was Maria. The force, energy, presence that animated this body will no longer be animating this body. All that will remain (and perhaps all that currently exists) of Maria will be in the stored memories of my friends, family, and acquaintances.

"My mother died over sixty years ago. Of those who knew her, I possibly carry the most defined image of her, the clearest feeling of her will, personality, and desires. I carry her instinct to guide me well into the world. She lives in me; I have become another vessel for her manifestation of life. Love is here, and it lasts beyond the final goodbye.

"I don't know how I am going to die," Maria said. "In preparation I strive for balance today; this could be the day. And then, I will no longer have consciousness to care what happens next. The ego that differentiates me will cease. The energy that I am entertaining at the time of my passing away will be sweeter or not so sweet, depending upon how I am now. So, I set aside time for stillness; it is a source of balance, resets the drives of everyday life; puts me in touch with the ease of contentment in the presence of just being. I practice not wanting to be otherwise; life is too precious."

Question for reflection: What enduring memories do you have of someone who has died but lives on in you?

Becoming a Seeker, Finding the Unexpected

When my mother was diagnosed with congestive heart failure in her early nineties and was given just months to live, she put the big question to my wife Cindy: What do you think will happen after I die? Our family was Jewish, but mostly by culture, and with little in the way of religious beliefs or spiritual exploration to fall back on, Mom struggled with the idea of where death would take her. Her questions became a quest for Cindy, who wound up trying to answer them by collecting stories from a range of wisdom traditions about death, the afterlife, and the transformations that death brings.

She published them later in a book called *The Wave and the Drop*, which takes its title from the simple Hindu story that gave my mother the most comfort in her last days. It imagines our lives as single drops of water thrown from the wave of Life. For a brief time, each drop has an individual life of its own. And then it falls back into the wave and the vaster sea of which it's a part. We arise from Life's great ocean, and to it we return.

Working on the book forced Cindy to wrestle with her own beliefs, fears, and hopes about life after this life, and she carried on her explorations after my mother was gone and the book was completed.

Cindy had her own urgent need to understand. After decades of environmental work, she has concluded that we humans are almost certainly among the hundreds of thousands of species on the brink of extinction as our planet warms beyond its ability to sustain us. And in the face of that, she feels the urgency of finding ways to comfort and guide people through the looming crisis, which she believes will plunge all of us into a world of suffering beyond what we've seen.

Her quest to understand life beyond these bodies has taken her into experiments with out-of-body experiences, research on near-death experiences, and into a series of conversations about the afterlife with a close friend. These conversations unfold as she writes questions to her friend, who died in 2017, and hears the answers in her mind. (She's published a small book of these "channeled" conversations called *Seven Questions About Life After Life*, and is at work on follow-ups.)

Cindy had experienced the mystical aspects of reality even as a child taking communion in the Catholic Church.

"I remember many times when I returned to the pew and knelt down to experience Jesus inside me, I encountered a brilliant white light, a white-out I called it," she says. "It only lasted a few seconds but it happened often. I never talked about it, but assumed everyone who received communion had the same experience. It's the most positive memory I have from that period of Catholic education. It might be called a peak experience, a mystical experience. I didn't have a name for it."

She left the church when she got older, rejecting the narrowness she perceived in its attitudes and putting her energies into social justice and environmental work. Then, when she was divorced from her first husband, she was also excommunicated. But as she worked to understand the stories of other cultures, she realized she also needed to revisit her own. And they looked substantially different from the 1950s Catholic-school version she had grown up with.

She was surprised to find that "the Story of Heaven went through a major revision that focused on how heaven was a place that welcomed everyone, where 'no sheep was considered lost,' and where each soul was beloved of God—in MLK's words, 'a member of the beloved community,' on earth and in heaven.

"The biggest surprise for me came when I found out that hell was no longer eternal," she says. "It was separation from God, self-imposed because of refusal to change bad behaviors. But angels or spirits were always sending out calls to join the community, and eventually many do. Leading Christian and Islamic theologians now subscribe to this version. As I described it to friends, 'Hell went poof.'"

The shift she discovered in the church of her childhood "was a microcosm of the change in my soul," she says. "Being able to embrace the wisdom of all the traditions"—including her own—"was so liberating for me." And the openness she felt drew her into her current explorations.

"After writing the revised Story of Heaven," she wrote in her journal, "I've had to adjust my mind and my heart to the core learning: You are so loved. Each of us is recognized as being within the One . . . I've been on a good path, but the horizon ahead just got more welcoming."

EXERCISE:

Revisiting Childhood Beliefs

If you've rejected or been rejected by the religion of your childhood, look to see what parts of yourself you might've left there and want to reclaim. Sometimes what we once rejected no longer stands. And sometimes the passionate literal belief of a child carries the seed of something we badly need in later life—faith or encompassing love or simple curiosity and openness to the power of the stories and rituals that are part of our inherited traditions.

Following the Truth that Takes Us Home

We don't know where our questions about eternity will lead us in later life. All we can do is follow them toward what rings true to our spirits.

I've been surprised by the turns in my own path as I've reached toward an understanding of the eternal and eternity. For years, particularly when I was a mathematician and space scientist, some equivalent of the Wave and Drop story worked for me. I saw myself dropping back into the immensity of All That Is after an incarnate journey in my body, not hoping or believing that my personality or individual soul would endure after I died.

Now, after more years of pondering and self-transcendent experiences, and undoubtedly influenced by what I've seen in Cindy, I've come down on the side of life after life. This life, I've come to believe, is a moral gymnasium and we are here to learn lessons of great import to us. After death, we review these lessons and our "experiences in the gym" so we can grow and develop from life to life.

My sense now is that Love and Light are not just New Age slogans but characteristics of what we will all experience when we die—an all-enveloping Love and a white-light experience that are part of our journey to life after life. It brings me peace to think of reuniting with loved ones who have gone before me.

At the same time, I've come to regard more and more places in my life as sacred spaces: the pillow where I lie in the morning, looking at the sleeping face of the person I love more than anything; the street corner where I talked to a neighbor; the desk where I sit listening to the worries of a friend whose test results frighten him; the chair where I sat beside my mother, trading rare and healing *I-love-yous* in the weeks before she died. My spirit has soared on trips through the world to places I consider holy and with which I feel a euphoric sense of connection. But increasingly I treasure the peace and stillness I find in being present every day with whatever comes and experiencing the life and bliss to be found there.

As I work to open to eternity in the time I have left, I take as my guide Rilke's poignant words: "Be patient toward all that is unsolved in your heart and try to love the questions themselves, like locked rooms and like books that are now written in a very foreign tongue. Do not now seek the answers, which cannot be given you because you would not be able to live them. And the point is, to live everything."

I don't hold up my beliefs as a model. But I hope they'll be the beginning of a conversation. Whether you agree or reject them out of hand, I hope they'll bring your own beliefs into sharp relief and let you see them more clearly.

EXERCISE:

Opening to Spiritual Possibilities

Any of the questions for reflection in the sections above can take you deeper into your conversation with the eternal. If you're a person who's turned away from the spiritual side of life, you may resist that exploration. But I hope you'll consider the possibility that it may yet hold something of value for you. My goal is not to steer you toward any particular paradigm, but to share with you what I've observed.

It's not unusual for people who have been humanists or atheists to emerge from adulthood into later life and realize that their perspectives have shifted. They have entered a new stage where new questions emerge, especially when their time is short: Is death really the end or is it a transition? If there is an afterlife, what is it like? Does my recent praying during later-life struggles imply that there is something or someone I am praying to? If so, what is this God like?

I've had many end-of-life discussions with people searching for a new understanding. I guided them with comments and questions like the ones below, which I recommend as starting points if you need them.

- You can choose to hold onto the story that when we die, we "fade to black" and disappear. But would you contemplate other stories, perhaps a story of establishing a relationship with the eternal?

- If you were to consider establishing a relationship with "something more," something greater than our individual lives, what form would it take and how would you cultivate it? Do you resonate at all with Joseph Campbell's thoughts about the eternal? Might they be something to explore?

People talk about having faith in the existence of the eternal, but I haven't had much faith in faith. Rather, I've relied on experience, the experience of love, wonder, beauty, compassion, and awe which began, for me, at age nine when I felt comforted and uplifted by the presence of the moon on the stoop of my home in Brooklyn—a feeling of connection that continues to the present day.

Might such experiences inform your own sense of life's mystery and its deeper dimensions?

There are no right answers; only answers that are right for you. If this search compels you, simply live the questions.

What We're Growing toward Is Peace

The reality and potential of later life is much larger and richer than we're commonly told. We can't push away decline and the certainty of our death, but with Death and our Wise Self as advisers, we can go beyond our sense of a bounded, separate self to a feeling of union with all else and feel the inner peace that is later life's most profound gift.

Peace comes when we let go of the sense that we are only losing things in later life and become more aware of what we're gaining—joy, resilience, gratitude and, most fundamentally, a growing ability to fall into the eternal now. Later life liberates us to live beyond our egos. We can allow ourselves to evolve instead of having to make things happen day-to-day, moment to moment. We can respond to the world and ourselves from a place of communion and wholeness rather than relying solely on agency and action. There is something peaceful and holy about assuming that what happens to us each day is sent to awaken our souls.

This feeling of peace allows us to realize that life is not about acquiring and accumulating things but about relationships and understanding. Our relationships during later life, more than ever, determine the quality of our lives. As we lose loved ones we ask: What now? Who am I? How do I live my life day-to-day? Do I risk reaching out for friendships and companionship? Or do I live in the past with my memories and wait for my life to wind down and run its course?

We may be severely tempted to disengage, yet when we allow peace to become the backdrop of life, moment by moment, we can move toward new and renewed relationships and even the possibility of companionship, comfort, and loving presence. We can be excited by life again, and discover that through new and renewed relationships we can be happy.

Peace rather than potential can be the emotional and spiritual ground of our lives. For me, that's meant that I've finally embraced who I am rather than feeling as if everything I am and have done is merely "spring training" for yet more doing, more accomplishment. When we quiet ourselves in these rich, blessed days of later life, we finally realize that what we've always been searching for outside ourselves lies within. As Rumi put it so beautifully: "I have been a seeker and I still am, but I stopped asking the books and the stars. I started listening to the teaching of my soul."

If only I had known how to allow and feel this peace so deeply when I was younger, I think sometimes. But it takes time and experience, love and loss, to know our own souls. It takes wisdom to see that, as May Sarton says, "Old age is not an illness, it is a timeless ascent. As power diminishes, we grow toward the light."

From our wisdom years we can bless the young—and each other—with the only advice we need to hear:

Know thyself. Love thyself. Accept thyself. After all, you are enough.

ACKNOWLEDGMENTS
With Gratitude

First, I am indebted to the older men and women I've known who have taught me so much about the blessings and burdens of life's last chapters. They have generously opened their hearts and allowed me to bear witness to their truths. Each of your experiences helped create this book.

My most heartfelt thanks go to Donna Frazier Glynn, whose wise counsel, skillful work, and immense dedication to *Our Wisdom Years* were invaluable. Donna clearly appreciated the book's importance and labored closely with me these many months to give it life. Simply put, she is a pleasure to work with and I offer my deepest gratitude to her.

To Jeff Herman, my literary agent, who, once again, expertly negotiated everything with Central Recovery Press (CRP) and found *Our Wisdom Years* just the home I wanted.

To Kirby Gann, who edited *Our Wisdom Years* with great skill thereby helping me create the best book I possibly could. Kirby's diligence—along with that of Valerie Killeen, CRP's managing editor; Patrick Hughes and John Davis in sales and marketing; Nancy Schenck, who did the final copy editing; and Marisa Jackson, the book's cover and interior designer—demonstrated clearly that this was their book, too.

To Cindy Spring, whose evocative personal story and profound insights were vital contributions to *Our Wisdom Years* and consequently to our understanding of later life. Bless her for seeing that this book is about love and gratitude, joy and forgiveness, loss and suffering, and opening to eternity. She knew that the book was also my attempt to make sense of my own later life and always supported this desire and need.

To my parents, Edward and Sylvia Garfield; and my in-laws Chick and Rita Centkowski, each of whom lived later life in a way that revealed the satisfactions and sorrows of growing old.

To Bella and Layla, who are both demonstrating that the lessons of aging are not only learned from humans. Their companionship is a much-appreciated reminder of the importance of love in daily life.

The only way I can adequately thank those kind souls who offered endorsements for *Our Wisdom Years* is to pay forward to others the kindness they showed me.

Special thanks to Kaushik Roy, Shanti Project's current executive director, for supporting both a founder's enduring love for and ongoing contributions to our beloved organization. Bless you and your entire team for caring so much about Shanti's welfare and the clients we serve.

Sincere admiration and respect for the thousands of Shanti Project volunteers, clients, staff, and board members for demonstrating daily that love heals.

The personal stories and insights given to me by Bharat Lindemood, Gina Belton, Micaela Salort Corazon, Judith Frank, John Amodeo, and Maria Straatman were wonderful contributions to *Our Wisdom Years*. My thanks to each of these wise ones for being there when I needed them.

Among older men and women and among those who live with and/or care for individuals of a certain age, there is so much of profound importance that people think and feel but have not yet spoken about in our families and friendship networks around the world. This creates a unique opportunity for *Our Wisdom Years* to be, in some small way, a voice for the dispersed and, too frequently, unheard aging community. If we listen, we will hear older people and their families, lovers, and friends, health professionals and volunteers say, "Something very important is happening among us, something fundamental to the way older people live fully, something that can teach us all how to go through life with joy, meaning, resilience . . . and few regrets."

RECOMMENDED READING

Introduction

Aging: The Fulfillment of Life
Henri J. M. Nouwen and Walter J. Gaffney, Image Books, 1976

Finding Meaning in the Second Half of Life: How to Finally, Really Grow Up
James Hollis, Gotham Books, 2005

On the Brink of Everything: Grace, Gravity, and Getting Old
Parker J. Palmer, Berrett-Koehler Publishers, 2018

Chapter One

Conscious Living, Conscious Aging: Embrace and Savor Your Next Chapter
Ron Pevny, Atria Paperback, 2014

Essential Spirituality: The 7 Central Practices to Awaken Heart and Mind
Roger Walsh, John Wiley and Sons, Inc., 1999

Life's Last Gift: Giving and Receiving Peace When A Loved One Is Dying
Charles Garfield, Central Recovery Press, 2017

Chapter Two

Living an Examined Life: Wisdom for the Second Half of the Journey
James Hollis, Sounds True, Inc., 2018

Living Your Unlived Life: Coping With Unrealized Dreams and Fulfilling Your Purpose in the Second Half of Life
Robert A. Johnson and Jerryl M. Ruhl, Jeremy P. Tarcher/Penguin, 2007

The Force of Character and the Lasting Life
James Hillman, Ballantine Publishing Group, 1999

Chapter Three

Awakening Joy: 10 Steps to Happiness
James Baraz and Shoshana Alexander, Parallax Press, 2012

The Happiness Curve: Why Life Gets Better After 50
Jonathan Rauch, Thomas Dunne Books, 2018

The Happiness Hypothesis: Finding Modern Truth in Ancient Wisdom
Jonathan Haidt, Basic Books, 2006

Chapter Four

Ageless Soul: The Lifelong Journey toward Meaning and Joy
Thomas Moore, St. Martin's Press, 2017

Memories, Dreams, Reflections
C.G. Jung, Vintage Books, 1989

Wise Aging: Living with Joy, Resilience, and Spirit
Rabbi Rachel Cowan and Dr. Linda Thal, Behrman House, 2015

Chapter Five

Forgiveness Is a Choice:
A Step-by-Step Process for Resolving Anger and Restoring Hope
Robert D. Enright, American Psychological Association, 2001

The Art of Forgiveness, Lovingkindness, and Peace
Jack Kornfield, Bantam, 2008

The Book of Forgiving:
The FourFold Path for Healing Ourselves and Our World
Desmond Tutu and Mpho Tutu, Harper Collins, 2014

Chapter Six

Gratitude
Oliver Sacks, Alfred A. Knopf, 2015

Gratitude Works!: A 21-Day Program for Creating Emotional Prosperity
Robert A. Emmons, Jossey-Bass Publishers, 2013

Thanks!: How Practicing Gratitude Can Make You Happier
Robert A. Emmons, Houghton Mifflin, 2008

Chapter Seven

Creating a Spiritual Legacy: How to Share Your Stories, Values, and Wisdom
Daniel Taylor, Brazos Press, 2011

The Legacy Guide:
Capturing the Facts, Memories, and Meaning of Your Life
Carol Franco and Kent Lineback, TarcherPerigree, 2006

Your Legacy Matters: Harvesting the Love and Lessons of Your Life
Rachael A. Freed, MinervaPress, 2013

Chapter Eight

Lovingkindness: The Revolutionary Art of Happiness
Sharon Salzberg, Shambhala, 2002

Real Love: The Art of Mindful Connection
Sharon Salzberg, Flatiron Books, 2017

The Mastery of Love: A Practical Guide to the Art of Relationship
Don Miguel Ruiz, Amber-Allen Publishing, 1999

Chapter Nine

Aging with Wisdom: Reflections, Stories, and Teachings
Olivia Ames Hoblitzelle, Monkfish Book Publishing Company, 2017

Cosmic Consciousness: A Study in the Evolution of the Human Mind
Richard Maurice Bucke, Martino Publishing, 2010

Religions, Values, and Peak Experiences
Abraham H. Maslow, Penguin Books, 1994

7 Questions About Life After Life: Book One, The Greater Reality Series
Cynthia Spring and Frances Vaughan, Wisdom Circles Publishing, 2019

The Essential Rumi
Translations by Coleman Barks with John Moyne, Harper Collins, 1995

The Five Stages of the Soul:
Charting the Spiritual Passages that Shape Our Lives
Harry R. Moody, Anchor Books, Doubleday, 1997

The Grace in Aging: Awaken as You Grow Older
Kathleen Dowling Singh, Wisdom Publications, 2014

The Perennial Philosophy
Aldous Huxley, First Harper Perennial Classics, 2009

The Power of Myth
Joseph Campbell and Bill Moyers, Anchor, 1991

The Varieties of Religious Experience: A Study in Human Nature
William James, Penguin Classics, 1982

The Wave and the Drop: Wisdom Stories about Death and Afterlife
Cindy Spring, Wisdom Circles Publishing, 2018

Walking Each Other Home: Conversations on Loving And Dying
Ram Dass and Mirabai Bush, Sounds True, 2018